Pain Or No Pain

The Chiropractic Connection
Dr. Micheline Côté DC

From the dictionary ...

chiropractor n.

One whose occupation is the practice of chiropractic.

chiropractic n.

A therapeutic system based primarily upon the interactions of the spine and nervous system, the method of treatment usually being to adjust the segments of the spinal column.

From Koine Greek etymology ...

cheir (χείρ) Definition: a hand

praktoros (πράκτοροσ) Definition: under the jurisdiction of

About the Cover ...

Diane Côté, the author's sister, took visual arts training at the University of Moncton in New Brunswick. While growing up in a chiropractic environment she developed a health consciousness that inspired the cover's illustration. She has named the picture "The Energy Connection" for its representation of universal and innate forces. Diane currently lives in Carpinteria, California with her husband, Jerry and children, Jules and Ali.

Published By: Kainos Enterprises
                  7777 Churchville Road
                  Brampton Ontario Canada L6Y 0H3

ISBN: 978-0-9685427-1-2

Erin Mills Optimum Health
3105 Glen Erin Dr. Suite 8
Mississauga ON L5L 1J3
905-828-2014
mjcote@bellnet.ca
www.pain-or-no-pain.com

Dedication

I would like to dedicate this book to my father,
Dr. Renaud Côté and my father-in-law, Dr. Fred Soloduka,
who are no longer with us.
They would have wholeheartedly approved this book
and its quest to disseminate the chiropractic story.

Contents

Connection Stories

Acknowledgments

First of all, I would like to thank Gary Carter for being the fuse that ignited this project, for his enthusiasm for this health care system that is chiropractic, for his patience and perseverance through sometimes difficult situations.

Next I would like to thank Wendy Carter, Gary's lovely wife, for putting my thoughts into words so competently and for all her hard work in researching the data. She is now a very knowledgable chiropractic expert.

I am grateful to my family, Steve, Julie and Max, for their encouragement and help with some of the passages in this book. Thanks, Max, for your input on Chapter 4!

Thanks also go to my sister, Diane, for her beautiful illustration for the front cover. She has put her heart and soul into this masterpiece and for that I am very pleased.

Finally, to the patients who have shared their stories with you, I wish to extend my gratitude. It was out of enthusiasm for chiropractic care and the desire to help their fellow man that they put effort and energy into this selfless act. They truly exemplify one of the quotes I live by, "A candle loses nothing by lighting another!"

Micheline

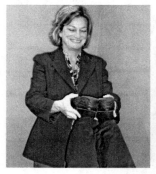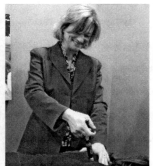

Dr. Micheline Côté with a patient.

Foreword

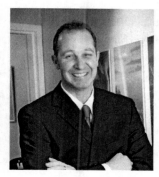

Dr. David Fletcher DC

There is an unfinished calling to serve within each of us. Some find a way to express their talents through paint and brush while others give speeches. Then there are the few who convey their gift through touch and the written word. I stumbled through my early years in practice searching for the ideal way to answer this calling. To my delight I found a community of like-minded professionals who would influence and enhance my perspective of health, healing, friendship and certainty. Dr. Côté was part of this group and her talents naturally positioned her as a skilled leader. She exuded an aura of calm wisdom that allowed all of us to ease into our lives and practices. You are about to read what have become important words and messages from a committed, loving and caring professional who has taken the time to listen and learn from her patients.

Micheline was nurtured in a family where healing, health and community were core values. This has translated into her practice and onto these pages. The stories that are told in this book are heard by chiropractors in every city and town, countless times a day. Our role is to share a message of wellness using our hands, our skills and Vis Medicatrix Naturae, "the healing power of nature". We work to unwind the damage that stress and traumas inflict on our neighbors. Spinal nerve tension exists in every age group and contributes to a loss of health and joy throughout the world. Micheline, or Miche, as she is fondly referred to, has collected and organized her healing experiences in an easy-to-read format so that the message of hope and healing through chiropractic can reach a broader and more necessary audience.

The healing message that is put forward in this book begins with the common theme that draws most people into our realm. We are all human after all and we experience our world, at times, through pain or symptoms. The joy of the chiropractic message is that it is not limited to therapy or pain management. In fact, this is only the starting point from which a health and wellness relationship can grow. Chiropractic adjustments are designed to tap into the inborn wisdom of the body and ignite the power that lies within. There is no one better at arousing this innate perfection than Micheline and as you read the stories within you will feel the admiration of her practice members.

Miche has written an important book that allows the individuals whose lives have changed to share their story. Enjoy the journey of learning and exploring as you read about these important transformations. In every one is a message that will change your life and the lives of those who you reach out to.

David

Dr. David Fletcher DC, FCCSS(C)
Clinician, lecturer and coach

Fletcher Chiropractic Clinic
1890 Glenview Rd., Pickering, Ontario L1V 1W8
www.docfletch.com

"The power that made the body, heals the body." This chiropractic statement has molded and nurtured generations of chiropractors and was instrumental in shaping the career of Dr. David Fletcher. Dr. Fletcher is widely recognized for his ability to communicate and teach students, patients and doctors about the power of chiropractic. He lectures extensively on the neurological aspects of natural healing and has pioneered the "nerve first" approach when examining and caring for patients. He was recently awarded the "Chiropractor of the Year" award for a prestigious chiropractic think tank and was featured on the cover of an international publication.

Introduction

Pain is one of our greatest enemies but also one of our best allies. For eons we have been attempting to minimize it in one way or another. In reality, pain is a symptom of a problem that has to be solved. It is our body's strategy to alert us to something wrong. Pain, temperature and touch sensors exist for that reason. It is not a mistake that we were equipped with them. They help us to survive.

This book addresses pain because it is a powerful motivator. Pain will kick us into action, incite us to seek treatment, urge us to click that mouse or pick up a book such as this one.

It is my goal as a chiropractor to make you look at pain differently and to not treat it as a mistake of the universe. It is an alarm system that helps you deal with crises. In a well functioning body with a well functioning nervous system pain always arises as the appropriate warning for a potentially damaging situation. For instance, if you put your hand on a hot stove you will get temperature and pain signals alerting you to respond immediately. This is what saves you from the catastrophic outcome that would occur otherwise.

Once you read this book you will understand more about pain and the reason for its existence. You will have strategies to deal with it and even eliminate it. You will also find that these strategies are not as elusive as you might think.

Don't just take my word for it. Read the words of the patients who have agreed to tell their *Connection Story*. These stories all come from the patient's perspective. I didn't coach them on what to say. I want these stories to be communicated because they will reach the hearts and minds of many. This cuts the chiropractor out of the process and simply flows from the patient's perspective to the prospective patient. I like that.

With these *Connection Stories*, some patients have their picture included to show they are real people. A few asked that their last name be reduced to an initial for privacy reasons. My comments after each one uses their stories to tell a story. They are as non-technical as I can make them, or else it would read something like this, "Pelvic and lumbar dyskinesia, subluxation of the right ilium, L5, C5, C1." and you would simply move on to the next page. I also have expanded their stories to the rest of my practice to let you know that these testimonies are not isolated events but occur on a day to day basis in a chiropractor's office. Notice too that these patients' care plans vary as to individual needs.

Life can be simpler than you believe or are led to believe. In my backyard I hang an empty blown up brown paper bag tied by a string from my patio umbrella. This simple technique drives away wasps. These insects are very territorial and they assume my brown paper bag is another wasp nest. It works wonderfully and we can enjoy our meals in peace outside. Many don't use this easy technique because they don't know about it. Instead they spray toxic substances to kill the wasps or use gooey, syrupy dishes to attract and trap them. Did you ever try cleaning these dishes after a few days? What a mess!

In similar fashion many don't seek out a chiropractor simply because they don't know much about what a chiropractor does. Instead they first try toxic solutions such as medication or even more drastic remedies that are less than practical like organ removal or alteration. The main objective of this book is to explain how most times there is a simple answer to a problem and that it can work in conjunction with your environment. The answer is chiropractic.

Before we go any further and to assist you in your reading, you need to realize that every field of knowledge does have its own language. Chiropractic is no different. Two key words used over and over are "misalignment" and "subluxation." They don't mean exactly the same thing but they are close.

Misalignment describes the state of position between two bones that are not lined up properly. Think in terms of watching a child stack blocks to build a tower that are not perfectly straight or walking on two patio stones that are not lined up correctly. Subluxation is a more precise word that includes the effects of the misalignment. One of the effects is the excessive wear and tear occurring between two misaligned bones. This causes degenerative changes and discomfort. But the most important consequence of subluxation is its affect on the nervous system. A chiropractor uses various tests to determine the extent of any of these effects. We'll talk more about these later.

Please be assured you don't have to brace yourself for a textbook sort of read. Just enjoy the information. Most of all develop a greater confidence in your body's ability to heal itself. The choice is yours. Option 1 is to continue in pain. Option 2 is to visit a chiropractor to deal with the cause of the pain. I know that after gaining more knowledge about how your body functions and how chiropractic works Option 2 will be a better choice. The famous entertainer, Madonna, travels worldwide with her many shows. Guess who she takes along — her own chiropractor! She has learned how beneficial chiropractic can be for her body.

Thought to Ponder:

Do sore thumbs really stick out?

"The doctor of the future will give no medicine but will interest his patients in the care of the human frame."

attributed to: Thomas Edison, Inventor

1

Connecting with the Doctor
How Smiley Faces Set Me on a Career Path

Many regarded my French Canadian father's profession as quackery back in the 1960s in Edmundston, New Brunswick. I consoled myself by the fact that others, particularly his patients, regarded him as a miracle worker. Renaud Côté was the third chiropractor to enter the province. Not many people knew much about this profession in New Brunswick at that time.

It is true my family was seen as a bit of an oddity initially. Since my father was the only chiropractor in town, we had to do a lot of explaining as we grew up. And yet my father was an excellent communicator. He built bridges with the community by being active in the Knights of Columbus. He was elected as a school board trustee and eventually became the board's president. It would have been hard to find someone in the city of Edmunston who didn't know my father. Over the years he helped a large percentage of the population with some of their health problems and thus gained the respect of his town.

Home Is Where My Heart Is

As a child growing up, I loved overhearing my father conversing, laughing and caring for his patients in the basement office of our home. He was very big on humor and had the most remarkable positive attitude I have ever observed. He believed it to be a great contribution to the overall healing process. He hung "keep smiling" signs all over his office. I can still visualize those little square cards posted everywhere.

My mother, Claudette, was always around as a full-time mom to keep our household running smoothly. She taught my family the love and art of good, nutritional cooking. She was an ardent fan of my father and his profession, initially working as his secretary. When my sisters and I came along, she decided it would be best to be replaced in the office as she had her hands full with us.

Chiropractic was not yet legislated in the province so my father became involved in the politics of it all, sitting on the first board of the New Brunswick Chiropractic Association to help his profession become established.

My father took care of the health of my sisters, Lise and Diane, and myself until adulthood. He firmly believed that the body could heal itself if the nervous system functioned well. He adjusted us regularly, particularly when we faced a health challenge.

Home Life and Our Health

In our home we very seldom visited a family doctor unless in an emergency with a broken bone. The only vaccination my father allowed us to have was a polio shot because it was a legal requirement for school attendance in those days. When I had a few bouts of tonsillitis, my father did not choose antibiotics nor the surgery approach even though it was very common at the time. He believed that if the spine is aligned properly, it would help the nervous system maintain a solid immune system which would not necessarily prevent but aid in dealing with sickness. The nervous system would communicate better with the immune system and the body would be protected efficiently. With this approach I retained ownership of my tonsils.

Another vivid memory I have is one day when looking outside from the upstairs window of our home I saw an ambulance arrive at our door. The attendants carried out a man on a stretcher. He was taken to my father's office downstairs. A little while later I saw this same man walking out the door on his own two feet! I didn't pay much attention to what my father told me about the adjustment he provided but it certainly worked in this gentleman's case. At such an early age I knew I had witnessed something special. This may have been my "aha!" moment in becoming a chiropractor myself.

My father also loved the independence and freedom his profession allowed. He could manage his own office by being able to choose the people he wanted to work with and set his own hours. The commute was about 30 seconds from the breakfast table to his office!

Through my teen years my father was very eager for me to follow in his footsteps as a chiropractor because he loved his profession so much. He often told me that there was no other profession that could give the kind of satisfaction that being a chiropractor gave. You could help people get well without drugs or surgery because their bodies work better.

My First Steps

Eventually I took the first step to enroll in the College St. Louis Maillet – a campus of the University of Moncton in Edmunston, New Brunswick – for a two-year diploma course in Health Sciences. (A three-year Bachelor of Science degree is now required.) This provided the prerequisite education for acceptance to the Canadian Memorial Chiropractic College (www.cmcc.ca). I started in 1978 in Toronto, Ontario. It was the only recognized chiropractic college in Canada back then. This four-year course was an arduous program that included many parallel courses to those a medical student faces to become a medical doctor.

My college years were ten months long instead of eight. We went to class from nine until four without "free" periods as it is today in most universities. We were fortunate to have great teachers that were borrowed from Sunnybrook Hospital and the University of Toronto's medical program to learn about the body. Neurological study was particularly intricate and emphasized since that is a chiropractor's ABC's. Also many hours were spent every year mastering the skills of adjusting spines and other joints.

Upon graduation in 1982, I returned home to New Brunswick and married a classmate, Steve Soloduka. We planned to return to Ontario to start our practices. My father wouldn't get his practice partner after all! We were married on September 18 – the same day chiropractic was founded in 1895. It was years later when we connected the dots and realized that our wedding day had taken place on the actual anniversary of chiropractic.

Living the Dream Together

I became an associate of Dr. Arnold Roper in Oakville for five years; Steve practiced with his chiropractor father in Toronto. I am so very grateful to Dr. Roper for all that I learned from him – running a business, managing people, educating patients and especially using the Activator technique for my patients. (More on that later.) He was an excellent, passionate role model teaching me a big portion of what I know today in my practice.

Steve eventually purchased the practice of a prominent Toronto chiropractor, Dr. Lloyd McDougall. I, in turn, purchased Erindale Chiropractic Clinic in 1987 in Mississauga, just a few miles west of Toronto, from two young chiropractors. They had built the practice from scratch and after three years decided to move out of the area. Lauren James, whose daughter's (Alison Hamouth) testimony appears later, was their assistant at the front desk and she remained in that position effectively as my right hand for five years. I work three days a week as I am also a mother to my delightful children, Julie and Max. I know they are becoming strong advocates of chiropractic even now as they reach adulthood. Who knows? Maybe they will eventually become chiropractors too.

In 2008 I downsized my business obligations by moving into a multi-discipline health care office at Erin Mills Optimum Health.

Through these years I have been extremely fulfilled by following my father's example and successfully treating many patients with numerous ailments – not just back and neck pain. I inherited his same passion for chiropractic along with his characteristic sense of humor; smiling is second nature to me. I firmly believe that my mission is to help restore good health to my patients.

Now It's All about Your Health Problem Story

My greatest desire is to help you get healthier. I think it is imperative that everyone understand what a chiropractor can do by gently adjusting spines. Your health can be greatly improved physically, mentally and emotionally as you instill these new patterns into your life. I know. I see it every day in my office.

You probably have regular check-ups or appointments with your family physician, dentist, eye doctor, hearing specialist, hair stylist and even a fitness centre to keep your body looking good and performing well. Why not add a chiropractor to your list? Isn't your nervous system just as important as your hair or teeth? Many people take better care of their car than their body and live long enough to regret the fact they can replace a car but not their body.

And People Just Like You

I have many interesting firsthand stories for you. It is very rewarding for me to witness my patients overcome their health problems and achieve better health with chiropractic care. My father was right when he said that no other profession in the world could equal the level of satisfaction one gets from helping a fellow human being in this way.

These anecdotes are not really miracle stories; although they may seem that way to the individual telling their own story. And until you understand a little of what is going on in their bodies, some of the accounts you are about to read may seem extraordinary – you can't make this stuff up! But I assure you these are real people who are describing real problems. I know Steve's practice is full of accounts like these too. My dad's and my father-in-law's storybooks would be even fuller. I am sure you will be encouraged and motivated by reading these BC & AC stories (Before Chiropractic and After Chiropractic). Most likely your experience could be added to this list if you gave chiropractic a chance.

The miracle is that our bodies have been wonderfully created in the first place. The body has an amazing power to heal and regulate itself. As chiropractors, we give the body a fighting chance by clearing away interferences in the nervous system. It is our responsibility to both find those interferences and correct them so that the body can work at its best. Resorting to prescription drugs and surgery should be the last resource rather than the first to tackle most health problems.

Enjoy a pleasant journey through my thoughts and experiences. My wish for you is to reach that "aha" moment and understand how easy it is to find relief and regain health. The choice to visit a chiropractor is yours. Pain or no pain – you make the connections.

Cancel the Surgery Please

Name: .... Uromi Fernando
From: .... Mississauga, Ontario
Treated for: ..... Lower Back Pain; Better Health
during Pregnancy; Headaches

"In late December of 1996 after my first child was born I experienced pain in my lower back. One day I went to the basement of our home to do the laundry. I was bending over to sort clothes and all of a sudden I found myself flat on my back. I tried to get up but couldn't walk. I managed to get my husband's attention who was upstairs. I got to a walk-in clinic and the attending doctor advised me that the pain was coming from my lower lumbar and that eventually I would need surgery. He gave me some medication to ease the pain and I went home.

Soon I became concerned about taking the medication as I thought I might be pregnant with my second child at the time. I took a pregnancy test and it was confirmed we were indeed expecting again. I decided I wasn't going to take any more of the medication. After a few days the pain went away.

A few years later we moved into a new house. My back pains started reoccurring until I couldn't get out of bed without help. I couldn't work. My husband called around to find a woman chiropractor in the area. He located Dr. Côté and an appointment was made. I told her about my first incident. She took some x-rays. I learned I had a deteriorating disk, probably from an injury incurred when young that I couldn't remember.

About six months later I discovered that I was pregnant with my third child. I was continuing to see Dr. Côté on a regular basis and it seemed that I wasn't as sick with this pregnancy as with my other two children. Dr. Côté recommended that I bring my baby in for a check-up after delivery because it can be such a traumatic experience for the child. I decided all three children should see her and I am so amazed after being on a maintenance program that they don't get sick very often. I wish I had realized that when my first two were younger, sick with colds and ear infections. As soon as they feel a cold coming on now they ask, "Can I go see Dr. Côté?" They are all very active children. When my two older daughters who are involved in sports have said that they don't feel quite right, I have questioned it; but upon visiting Dr. Côté we have learned that their bodies are out of alignment in some way. Today I don't question; I make the appointment. We don't see our family doctor very often any more.

As to my own original health issue I have had no recurring, long term problems except when I tried skating once again or when I fell downstairs holding my baby. I used to have headaches when I was young but I don't suffer with them any more.

I highly recommend Dr. Côté to others. My husband has been visiting her for the past year. A friend at age 65 fell and injured his shoulder. She is helping him. Some people are afraid of manual adjustment – a method Dr. Côté doesn't use. Others only go once or twice to her office and that doesn't give enough time for proper healing.

I am very upset with our current health care system since our government no longer subsidizes chiropractic care. Doctors do have a place but both professions need to work together.

My youngest is now six and I am very pleased and comfortable with Dr. Côté's monthly service for my whole family."

Comments:
Uromi is the perfect example of how to keep your family healthy with a chiropractic lifestyle. After relief from a nasty lower back problem she had during her pregnancies she was interested in this drug free, gentle approach for her family's well being especially after realizing that such care helped with more than just back pain.

Her three girls have benefited tremendously by her decision. Through the years we have cared for them through colds, earaches, coughs, fevers, falls, postural problems, aches and pains. Many times adjustments replaced painkillers, antibiotics and puffers given too regularly to children before trying natural approaches.

Her husband has also benefited from chiropractic care for a toe pain problem that had been diagnosed as gout. After only a few adjustments we are realizing that it may have been a toe misalignment causing the pain. It went away after the toe was adjusted and the pain doesn't seem to be coming back.

Care Plan:
I saw Uromi three times a week initially. After four weeks we were able to decrease the frequency of visits gradually to once a month.

Connection Story

Does This Story Qualify as a Miracle Cure?
Name: .... Jo-Anne H.
From: .... Etobicoke, Ontario
Treated for: .... Fibromyalgia; Carpal Tunnel Syndrome

"I began Chiropractic adjustments with Dr. Steve Soloduka (Dr. Côté's husband) in January 2008 and within three months using the gentle Activator adjustment approach, I had the following improvements in mobility and pain management.

In three weeks the circulation in my right hand was improving for the swelling was decreasing and the colour of my hand was turning from white back to pink. Within three months, the swelling in my right hand had gone completely and I was able to straighten my hand with feeling in the tips of my fingers returning. My middle left finger was no longer clawing. The swelling in my feet had gone down and I could wiggle my toes. The muscles in my neck were not so knotted and I was able to move my head from left to right; whereas before I was moving my whole body. I had been beyond feeling in that area. The numbness of toes, swelling of ankles and knees were gone!

I am now walking straight and tall, no longer needing a cane for balance or a wheel transport chair on rainy days. The restricted movement of my neck, inability to raise arms above shoulder height, lower back and restless leg pain have been eliminated. I am also sleeping in my bed through the night with the use of a memory pillow – prior to treatment I normally slept in a winged chair. My hands are no longer swollen, movement of fingers are no longer restricted and they no longer curl towards the palm.

Although diagnosed with Carpal Tunnel Syndrome, my neurologist has postponed surgery until further observation can be made. My previous diagnosis of having Fibromyalgia is now under question as trigger points are no longer present when examined by my Rheumatologist.

Based on my personal experience with chiropractic care, I recommend that individuals regardless of current health situation, age or life circumstances include a Doctor of Chiropractic as part of their health care provider and wellness team.

Thank you Dr. Soloduka for giving me my life back!"

Comments:
After 25 years in practice, it still humbles me to witness the awesome healing powers of a chiropractic adjustment. Improving health and

improving quality of life is what chiropractic is all about. I am happy for Jo-Anne regaining her health in such a short period of time. My only regret is that more people have yet to discover the awesome healing potential of chiropractic.

From the heart, Dr. Steve Soloduka

Care Plan:

Jo-Anne was seen three times a week initially for six weeks, then twice a week for eight weeks and once a week after that.

Connection Story

Is Benjie Kidding?

Name: .... Benjie Caluag
From: .... Mississauga,
Ontario
Treated for: .... Hiccups; Plantar
Fasciitis

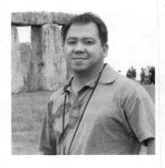

"My particular ailment is probably the most interesting case that Dr. Côté has ever treated. About two years ago I started suffering with very intense, continuous hiccups. I had problems with breathing and it was even difficult to eat. It was hard to do my job properly or anything else with this constant annoyance. My doctor couldn't solve my problem; a specialist took x-rays, a scan and I went for an MRI. I was prescribed pills for asthma and even tranquilizer pills with no improvement. I really felt miserable for one year.

One day a friend suggested that I visit Dr. Côté's office. I agreed since my insurance covered the costs. Dr. Côté gave me some tests and adjusted me three times that first week on my neck and chest. I realized that my hiccups were not as intense as before. After a month and reducing my appointments to once a week my hiccups had subsided. We were all surprised and I was delighted. I visit her office once every three months now because if I don't the hiccups return.

Dr. Côté has helped with other minor problems such as a painful heel called Plantar Fasciitis that was very hard to walk on about a year ago. That problem has gone now for which I am very grateful as well.

I have recommended Dr. Côté's services to others and I am pleased that they have taken my advice."

Comments:

When we received the call from one of our patients about Benjie's hiccups, I was a bit surprised because I had not heard of such a thing as continuous hiccups for a long period of time. This condition may sound a bit trivial to you, but when I saw Benjie we struggled through the consultation as he was out of breath and constantly interrupted by the hiccups. Imagine trying to fall asleep or even relaxing with this condition!

Hiccups are contractions of the diaphragm. Since the diaphragm has a nerve supply and chiropractic relieves nerve system interferences or disturbances I decided to accept Benjie's case on a trial basis.

I adjusted Benjie's cervical (upper) spine primarily but also his rib cage, sternum and xyphoid process. He responded beautifully to chiropractic care and we were both amazed and pleased.

Worthwhile to note is that once when Benjie was feeling great and too busy to come in, his hiccups redeveloped, so we figured that maybe because of his lifestyle it was better to check him every few months to make sure he didn't get any recurrences of this nasty problem.

Later on when Benjie developed Plantar Fasciitis, adjusting his heel and foot was very helpful. We often get terrific results with foot problems when there are misalignments in the bones of the foot.

Care Plan:
Benjie came to my office three times a week for a month, then once a week for a few more weeks and now once every three months.

Thought to Ponder:

**What happens when you get half
scared to death twice?
Are you then one quarter alive?**

**"Inflammation is the flame which
cleanses the body."**

Hippocrates, Father of Medicine

2

Connecting with Pain

How Pain Can Be Your Friend

All of a sudden in the middle of the night the smoke alarm goes off in your house. You don't run to take the battery out of the alarm to stop the annoying sound. You take proper action; upon smelling smoke you get up and call 911; you find your family members and leave immediately. Firemen arrive to extinguish the fire and save all that can be saved. Fire investigators determine the cause of the disaster. Was it the wires, the furnace, gas pipes, the electrical switches, the fireplace, an appliance? It could be many things.

Similarly, pain is like that smoke alarm. Unfortunately in our society, many people don't handle pain the way they should. Instead they subdue it, mask it, or try to ignore it. Pain killers are one of the biggest money makers for the pharmaceutical companies today. Billions of dollars are spent on an approach that can be downright dangerous to you much like the fire burning in your house. The right solution must be found.

More Than Putting Out Fires

Initially chiropractic care is like the firemen arriving at the scene and putting out the fire. That is in fact why most people consult with us to put out the fire of pain. Within a month most "fires" are put out for our patients, but there is damage left behind that can be helped with further care. We give this option to our patients. The body repairs many damaged tissues if the nervous system is functioning at its peak; therefore continuing chiropractic care will help.

Instead of waiting for the fire to spark, imagine if fire inspectors were sent in to evaluate the safety of your house, to check out all the things that can go wrong. That is exactly where our chiropractic profession shines the most. We serve as inspectors to find problems before they flare up. We have technology to measure nerve activity, temperature control of skin, heart rate variability in addition to joint movement tests that can signal a problem before any pain occurs. Chiropractors can evaluate how well you are functioning even before you feel any discomfort.

The Many Faces of Pain

You may have experienced various kinds of pain in your life from bumping your head on an open cupboard door to breaking your leg in a car accident. A misalignment in your body can cause different aches depending on which nerve fibers are affected. Some patients have excruciating pain from the distressed nerve while others have minor ache, numbness or skin sensitivity in the area.

Whispering Pain

Very often pain can start gradually instead of stabbing all of a sudden. The pain whispers before it shouts. When you first notice a twinge of discomfort in your body, do you hope that it will just disappear on its own? Be aware that this is a built-in warning system announcing that there is a problem. Often people treat pain as an inconvenience and do not fully appreciate its function. As previously mentioned you wouldn't just turn off a smoke alarm in your house before finding the cause of the smoke in the first place. You don't put duct tape over an oil light flashing in your car to make the glare go away without checking your oil first. You know that would be stupid. In much the same way, pain is your warning light or sound alarm to a problem. It's always best not to ignore it.

Pain Can Get Too Normal

If pain is habitual or long lasting (over three months in some descriptions) it is called "chronic" pain. It may come and go, start off mildly or be quite debilitating. This type of pain can result in depression, insomnia, exhaustion, worry, emotional stress, even weight loss or gain. All these can, in turn, lead to their own disorders such as stomach ulcers, addiction to pain killers, or erratic immune response, just to name a few. Learning to live with the pain is obviously not a good option especially when taking earlier action could help you recover faster.

It saddens me that so many of my patients have put up with a lot of unnecessary discomfort throughout the years. They could have put aside their misconceptions about chiropractic care and gained quick, easy relief from their suffering earlier on if only they had sought help sooner. Also, pain is intensified by fear and anxiety. You may be fearful because you do not understand what is happening to your body. When apprehension takes control it sometimes seems much easier and safer to just do nothing.

Chiropractic care is safer than pain killers, muscle relaxants and surgery. The results are more predictable. You do not know in advance how you will react to a prescription drug. Check out the numerous television commercials advocating a particular medication and notice the long list of side effects that are always attached. Why not try chiropractic first? This safe natural course of action should be considered before more invasive and possibly damaging procedures or medication. Dealing with a chronic problem almost always ends up taking longer than an acute one. The sooner you address your problem the faster it will respond. Everyone is different and will react at varying speed. As you read on you will understand this process better.

Radiating or Referred Pain

I can't help but marvel at how our bodies have been created. If you come to my office and complain of a pounding headache, don't be surprised when I find that the cause is a pinched nerve in your neck. Yes, I know you would think that the problem would be in your head.

Radiating pain can be felt at a location some distance away from the cause of the pain. For instance, leg pain (or sciatica) can be caused by nerve compression or irritation in the lower back; left arm pain may occur when you have heart problems; and you can have knee pain sometimes from an underlying foot or ankle problem.

No Pain or Not So Much

Please don't assume that everything is fine if you have no pain. Absence of pain doesn't necessarily mean the absence of a problem. Too frequently we have heard of a person dying suddenly and unexpectedly from a heart attack. Often no pain was felt before that catastrophic event.

Consider a health problem as an iceberg. Pain is represented by the tip of this iceberg – the part out of the water, the part you feel. The bigger part of the iceberg hidden under the water represents the rest of the problem. When you experience pain it is usually a small part of what is wrong.

Spinal nerve stress can build slowly and gradually without our awareness. People lead very busy lives with little time to pay attention to their bodies and how they function. Regular chiropractic care will prevent the occurrence of misalignments that can cause health problems and pain by detecting and correcting them sooner.

The Gift of Pain

Dr. Paul Brand, author of *The Gift of Pain*, recounts a story of four-year old Tanya who lived her life without pain. She had a "rare genetic defect known informally as 'congenital indifference to pain.' She was healthy in every respect but one: she did not feel pain. Nerves in her hands and feet transmitted messages about changes in pressure and temperature – she felt a kind of tingling when she burned herself or bit a finger – but these carried no hint of unpleasantness. Tanya lacked any mental construct of pain. She rather enjoyed the tingling sensations, especially when they produced such dramatic reactions in others."[1] Her desperate parents too often contended with Tanya's bizarre ways such as biting off her finger tip and playing with the oozing blood. She did not limp when she twisted her ankle or when her foot became infected from stepping on a nail or thumbtack which she did not bother to pull out. Unfortunately, there wasn't much that could be done for this little girl. Eventually she had to be institutionalized. Both of her legs had to be amputated; most of her fingers were gone; her elbows were often dislocated; ulcers covered her hands and amputation stumps; and due to her chewing habits her tongue was lacerated and scarred. What a sad life!

So what is this enemy we call "pain?" Britannica defines pain as "a complex experience consisting of a physiological and emotional response to a noxious stimulus. Pain is a warning mechanism that protects an organism by influencing it to withdraw from harmful stimuli; it is primarily associated with injury or the threat of injury."[2] The Merriam-Webster Dictionary reports that it is "a basic bodily sensation induced by a noxious stimulus, received by naked nerve endings, characterized by physical discomfort (as pricking, throbbing, or aching), and typically leading to evasive action."[3] Simply put by the Cambridge Dictionary, it is "a feeling of physical suffering caused by injury or illness."[4]

Unlike Tanya's sad life, we should be very grateful when we experience pain for it leads us to protective action. Pain safeguards our body and motivates us to find a solution sooner than later. Pain is really more a friend than an enemy. Also just making the pain go away artificially is not a good solution since there is an underlying problem. You need pain to nudge you toward a positive solution – not toward a pill bottle.

Will It Hurt?

Now that we understand pain, do you need to have more pain to get out of pain? Some people say "no pain, no gain." But is that really true? Could something gentle, pain-free and safe really work?

I can tell you that most new patients visiting my office are anxious about chiropractic care. They think it will be painful and dangerous. I am always amazed at that and my patients are even more surprised after their first adjustment realizing how comfortable and gentle it was. They seem relieved. Most leave with a smile and come back much calmer for their second visit.

Different Techniques Available for Your Comfort

Chiropractic care like medicine has progressed tremendously over the past century. Many new exam procedures and approaches for correction of spinal problems have been developed to improve accuracy, safety and comfort. Some of these techniques utilize instruments that deliver the force that is needed to move a vertebrae or a bone. The one I use is called "Activator Methods" and its instrument, the "Activator." I find it works best for me and my patients. I trained after graduating from college to learn this skill so I can provide very effective and safe care for the patients I see. It is a very individual choice, much the same as an artist would pick water color as opposed to acrylic for artistic expression. A technique, regardless of the delivery, should be a means to properly align the body's structure thus ending up with a better functioning nervous system.

Activator Methods

The Activator Methods were developed in the late 1960s to improve the comfort and specificity of the chiropractic adjustment. The use of the Activator tool is helpful in determining what needs to be adjusted and what doesn't. The Activator tool is an instrument about six inches (20 cm) long. It has a rubber tip at one end along with an internal adjustable spring mechanism which presets the applied force. It is held by the hand and squeezed to deliver a force. You can precisely apply the instrument to a location on a bone (point of contact) and direct the force in any chosen path. In fact, the force is delivered so quickly (1/200 to 1/300 of a second) that the brain doesn't have time to register the feeling of the thrust; so it doesn't hurt. All you notice is a clicking sound and a slight pressure at the point of contact of the instrument.

It took 40 years to get the Activator technique to the refined state it is at today. There were 15 years of scientifically monitored clinical trials. The latest advances in orthopedic science along with the intricate subject of neurology were considered. Since the places where the bones join are critical, careful measurements to understand proper alignment came into play. Today over 35,000 chiropractors have been trained in the use of this method. The Activator technique stands out as the second most widely used technique after the basic procedure taught in our colleges. I am one of about 500 chiropractors worldwide who is qualified to teach the use of this remarkable skill. Training seminars for chiropractors and chiropractic students happen most weekends in one city or another throughout our continent and now abroad. Recently Internet online education has been added to help chiropractors in remote areas train in the technique.

Some patients, during the initial stages of care, do feel a bit out of sorts while their body is returning to good health. I warn them of this possibility. This period is usually short in duration, less than a week, and mild in nature. There have been less than a handful of patients I recall not improving with the appropriate amount of care. Some of these special cases I have referred elsewhere to other health care providers. Others who didn't have the desired response quit care too soon to achieve the needed correction.

Is It Safe?

You need to know if chiropractic is harmful to the body initially or over time. You may have read or heard a story in the news questioning chiropractic care. Of course, the reason these stories hit the news is that they are so very rare whereas similar sad occurrences happen every day in other health care contexts. However, there is little or no scientific evidence to suggest that chiropractic is a risky choice.

An extensive seven-year study based on a large number of cases was recently published in the medical journal, *Spine*. Dr. J. David Cassidy (senior scientist at the Toronto Western Research Institute, Health Care and Outcomes Research Division) concluded that "the risk of stroke was about the same after seeing a chiropractor or a family doctor for patients presenting with neck pain ... people who visit chiropractors for a neck adjustment are no more likely to suffer a stroke than when treated by members of any other medical profession"[5]

Based on other scientific studies, we have learned that there isn't enough evidence to support that chiropractic adjustments can cause a stroke or damage to the vertebral artery. The risk of stroke has been proven identical under the care of a chiropractor and a medical doctor – less than one in one million. Dr. Scott Haldeman, a world leading neurologist and chiropractor from Santa Ana, California, stated in 2002, "Based on the scientific literature, the risk of stroke should be considered a rare, random and unpredictable complication associated with cervical adjusting." (www.spine-health.com.)

Why Is My Liability Insurance Much Less?

In addressing the question of the safety of chiropractic care consider this. I pay far less money for my chiropractic malpractice insurance premiums than a medical doctor pays. Why? The insurance companies set the premium rates according to the number of incidents that occur. If there were more problems caused by the chiropractic profession than other health professions, then it would follow that our premium rates would be just as high to cover the legal costs of malpractice law suits. Clearly, our chiropractic patients very seldom find fault with our care.

A few of my patients are medical doctors and I am delighted to have you read a recommendation from Dr. Gillian Brakel appearing later. She believes this science has a valuable place in our health care system.

Beyond Pain

August 4, 2008 marked a very exciting day for Canada. It was during the 29th Olympiad in Beijing, China and Canada earned 4 medals. Karen Cockburn from Toronto, Ontario won a silver medal in trampoline. In an interview after receiving her award, it was learned that her husband, Mathieu Turgeon, is also a master of this sport for he won a bronze medal in Sydney in 2004. He has since retired from this type of competition and graduated from Canadian Memorial Chiropractic College. He was so impressed at how chiropractic care helped his career that he decided to become one.

Lance Armstrong, famous cyclist racer, recommends chiropractic, "The team wasn't just riders. It was the mechanics, masseurs, chefs, soigneurs and doctors. But the most important man on the team may have been the chiropractor."

In 1988 in the summer Olympics in Seoul, South Korea, American Greg Louganis, winner of two gold medals previously, was performing in the diving competition. Unexpectedly, he hit his head on the board during one of his dives. A chiropractor quickly adjusted the misalignment found in his spine. This enabled him to continue on to win his third gold medal.

Do you want to be a good golfer? Tiger Woods says, "Being a chiropractic patient has really helped me immensely … lifting weights and seeing a chiropractor on a regular basis has made me a better golfer. I've been going to a chiropractor for as long as I can remember. It's as important to my training as practicing my swing."

Another World and Olympic Champion, Dan O'Brien, who won gold in 1996 in the decathlon, fully supports chiropractic service for he says enthusiastically, "If not for chiropractic, I would not have won the gold medal!"

The Athletes

Most athletes are very highly respected in our society; they achieve amazing feats of performance with their bodies. Many consult chiropractors on a regular basis so that the body can function at its full potential. These athletes would not subject their bodies to a science that doesn't get results and isn't safe. Chiropractic care helps them improve performance. When an injury does occur, they are able to return to competition faster; but more importantly, the athlete's nervous system is free of interference so that all messages transmitted to muscles and organs are clear. There is no cheating from body enhancing drugs as it is a natural intervention. Cortisone shots will dull the pain and reduce inflammation but like medication they can't help the underlying problem. Isn't your body as important as that of an athlete? And it might even enhance your performance in the workplace, in your family life, in any social activity because your body is truly operating at its best just as these well known athletes experience.

Connection Story

Where One Medical Doctor Turns for Help

Name: .... Dr. Gillian Brakel
From: .... Oakville, Ontario
Treated for: ..... Neck Pain with Neck Muscle
Spasms; Headaches

"I had been suffering from a long-standing neck problem for about ten years which caused headaches from neck muscle spasms. I had seen quite a few people with their various techniques of acupuncture, physiotherapy, and manual adjustment through chiropractic but these treatments didn't last. Besides it was getting expensive.

My parents had become patients of Dr. Côté who used a different technique called the Activator method. I made an appointment and she encouraged me to stick it out with her for a few months. She thought my neck was misaligned which caused the muscles to go into a spasm. She explained that this might have been due to stress or poor posture. I visited her office once a week for about two months and then this routine was reduced. She didn't encourage me to come back more often if it was not needed. This was about eight or nine years ago and since then the pain is gone except for a couple of months during my pregnancies. I continue to see her once every two months. My husband is a patient as well for his knee and back pain. He was quite a skeptic initially because of previous experiences but he feels results after being adjusted by Dr. Côté and will make an appointment immediately when he notices alignment is needed.

In my opinion chiropractic is excellent for neck or back pain and even knee pain. There is always the controversy between my profession of physicians and Dr. Côté's as a chiropractor as to how much treatment is appropriate. It's just a difference in philosophy but chiropractic can be a beneficial complementary health care system and can add to a patient's quality of life without using prescription or over-the-counter medicines. I have referred many of my patients to Dr. Côté. Her training is excellent and she seems to have a sixth sense to be able to pick up on problem areas and get to the root of them. I am all for finding the root of the problem rather than just masking it with medications. Dr. Côté's vocation is not just a job to her; she is genuinely concerned about her patients' well being. I am very happy to continue to refer people to her."

Comments:

Gillian is the daughter of a good friend of mine. I was seeing her mom as a patient for a while and she advised Gillian to come visit me when she was experiencing neck and headache problems. She also suffered from lower back pain and was diagnosed with a bulging disc causing pain for one year. Asthma symptoms appeared during the past three years.

I have to admit her lower back problem turned out to be a breeze to solve as compared to her neck problem. Through two pregnancies she did not have much lower back pain. Her regular chiropractic care was most likely helpful in that respect.

Her neck problems were a little more stubborn as every stress seemed to bring on a new bout. Adjustments were helpful but her neck pain came back when she was again under stress. Gillian is now much better thankfully and experiences only occasional neck pain between her bimonthly visits. Nevertheless, being a doctor with two young children does add an unusual amount of stress in her life.

Care Plan:

Gillian visited me a couple of times a week to begin with, then once a week for two months and now she comes once every two months.

Connection Story

Put on a Happy Face

Name: .... Glenna Somerville
From: .... Mississauga, Ontario
Treated for: ..... Facial Neuralgia (pinched nerve in neck); Lower Back Pain

"A few years ago I went for my six-month dental appointment. Everything was fine. The following Sunday I was invited to a friend's home for dinner. During dinner I had a terrible ache on the left side of my face which felt like an abscessed tooth. I had such intense pain I had to leave for home.

The pain was on the whole left side of my face which made my left eye quiver and my ear ache. I walked the floor in agony all night and went back to my dentist the next morning. X-rays were taken with no problem found with my teeth. My dentist diagnosed the pain as neuralgia and said the pain would eventually go away on its own. It was a pain that would hit suddenly, last anywhere from ten minutes to almost half an hour. I couldn't eat or drink anything that was the slightest bit warm such as tea.

I went to my doctor the same afternoon and she also diagnosed it as neuralgia. I was given some medication but it didn't do anything for the pain. A few days later the doctor referred me to a neurologist. He did a neurological exam, giving me the same diagnosis as the dentist and my own doctor – neuralgia (a disorder of nerves responsible for sensing touch, temperature, pressure and pain sensations in the facial area from the jaw to the forehead). They each said it would go away on its own, but there was no time limit given.

After some six weeks of severe pain, very little sleep, and lots of tears, I was sent to the neurologist for a second visit. He said to give it another week and if the pain was still as intense, he said, 'We'll have a CAT scan done and take it from there.' Whatever that meant!

A friend of mine asked me if I'd spoken with Dr. Côté, as I'd been going to her for a number of years. I never gave a thought to calling her, as I really didn't associate the chiropractor with the pain in my face. In desperation, I called Dr. Côté, in tears, and she was kind enough to see me right away.

On seeing me, she told me I looked terrible. (I sure did with no sleep and terrific pain for six weeks!) Dr. Côté did her usual exam and diagnosed my problem as a pinched nerve in my neck, the nerve that affects the complete left side of the face and head. I told her about being diagnosed with neuralgia and she explained that neuralgia is caused by a nerve being inflamed because it is pinched. She said it would take about eight visits. Once the nerve was unpinched it would take about a week for the inflammation to disappear. Dr. Côté gave me the first treatment right then and I had six more visits. After each visit the pain was less and less until after the seventh visit the pain was completely gone.

I happened to meet my neurologist about a month later and he commented on how well I looked and wanted to know how long it took for the pain to go away on its own. I told him I couldn't take the pain any longer and had taken it upon myself to see my chiropractor. I explained what Dr. Côté did for me and he was very pleased I'd gone to her. I am forever grateful to Dr. Côté and will always remember that chiropractors don't just treat back pain."

Comments:

When I first met Glenna, she could hardly walk because of the most acute sciatica problem (pain down one leg) I had ever seen. Fortunately she responded well to chiropractic care and was herself again in four weeks. After that experience I recommended that we check her every few months and did so for many years. Her leg problem has never returned. A few years ago, though, she did suffer from an acute bout of facial neuralgia (face pain) that was so severe she could not even sleep, talk or think straight. She had missed a few appointments when she finally called to ask my opinion. I thought we had a very good chance of helping her so she came into the office. She had a few weeks of adjustments until her pain went away. She had seen some neurologists before that understood what her problem was; however they only had muscle relaxants, tranquilizers and pain killers as an answer. This past year, Glenna began experiencing shoulder pain that was quite incapacitating. She is nearly back to normal from an ailment that can be sometimes very finicky to resolve. Glenna and I have been partners in her health care program for a long time now – successful with every difficulty that has arisen. She is now 80 years young!

Care Plan:

When Glenna first came to see me for her sciatica problem, she was scheduled three times a week and was fine after six weeks. Her facial neuralgia resolved in three weeks with three visits a week. Now I see her once every two months.

Connection Story

From Terrible to Terrific!

Name: .... Grazyna Malas
From: .... Mississauga, Ontario
Treated for: ..... Migraines; Back Pain; Depression;
                    Hand Pain

"I just didn't know where to turn next. I had so many health issues bothering me for several years such as migraines, back pain, inability to move my hand, and a terrible disposition which could have been depression. I was seeing a chiropractor who was using a manipulation method which sometimes made me worse. There was no explanation or plan of treatment. My muscles were so tense that every time I went I ended up suffering with another migraine headache.

Almost two years ago my husband's friend recommended trying Dr. Côté. When I arrived in her office I was actually crying because of all my various pain problems. I didn't know what the matter was with my body.

Dr. Côté x-rayed me and gave me a special test to measure the tension in my muscles called a Surface EMG. Treatment started; she had an exact plan in place. I met with her three times a week which program gradually lessened as the weeks went by. My situation was so unusual it took quite a while to isolate all the individual problems but the different hot points are becoming more obvious with only one out of two areas still flaring up.

Last month the measurement test was repeated and much to our surprise the results showed incredible improvement! Dr. Côté thought that her device was broken as I had sailed off the chart. I sit at a computer most of my day and so the upper part of my spine is not in good shape. My migraines have subsided in intensity and occur less frequently. I look forward to the day when my health is completely restored.

I definitely recommend Dr. Côté and her services to others!"

Comments:

Grazyna visited my office a few years ago with a complaint of neck stiffness that had been bothering her for about three years. Her symptoms were worse at night and more particularly with stress. She had suffered with chest pain a few years previously – a symptom that can be quite unnerving, adding to someone's stress level at the best of times.

Her x-rays revealed a significant deviation to the left of her thoracic (chest area) and cervical (neck) spine which could easily affect her rib cage and neck alignment resulting in the symptoms she was experiencing. Her adjustments were mainly for her upper spine and rib cage. She seemed to respond well to that approach. A pre and post Surface EMG showed tremendous improvement. This test is an indication of nervous system balance through a measurement of electrical activity of the spinal musculature.

However encouraging that was, Grazyna was still experiencing some neck discomfort from work-related stress. Sometimes I find mental stress can be just as disturbing to the spinal alignment as physical trauma. In Grazyna's case stress seems to be a very significant irritant.

Care Plan:
Grazyna met with me three times a week initially for six weeks. We decreased her visits to her current status of once every six weeks.

Earlier Is Better

Name: .... Doug Fairley
From: .... Windsor, Ontario:
Treated for: ..... Lower Back Pain;
                   Plantar Fasciitis

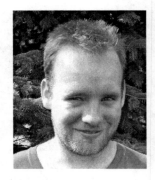

"No, I really didn't want to make an appointment with a chiropractor due to preconceived notions about what chiropractors do such as quick maneuvers with the body. I was apprehensive. I had temporarily moved to Brampton. I had periodically experienced lower back pain for the past few years but now it was amplified to the point that I wasn't sleeping at night. My new landlord suggested I see his chiropractor, Dr. Côté, who used a gentle method with an instrument known as an Activator. Being in my early 20s I knew I needed to try something and so I made the appointment. I had not seen my family doctor about this condition previously nor was I taking Tylenol to help with the pain.

The initial testing with Dr. Côté revealed that there was uneven electrical activity in my lower back muscles. This could have been most likely related to my pain. She treated various spots with her Activator and I had relief for about a day. I agreed to see her three times a week and after each visit the pain did not return as quickly. Appointments have been spread out to two and three week periods and I am gradually getting better. I did have a few other minor issues, such as a heel problem, which were helped. I now understand the healing process better and on a scale of 1-10, I am at 8 or 9. I look forward to a repeat test in a month or so for comparison.

I do recommend Dr. Côté's services sometimes to my friends, but unfortunately like me most of them are hard to convince."

Comments:

Doug came to my office initially for lower back pain which had been relatively minor for five years. It wasn't interfering with his activities so he endured it. A particularly bad bout of it along with some friends' encouragement was finally enough motivation to pursue chiropractic care.

Upon examination I noticed a significant lean of his spine to the left probably from an uneven pelvis shifting his weight distribution – and you guessed it – heavier on the left. As a result of this he was also

Connection Story

starting to feel left heel pain. After a few weeks of care adjusting his lower back and left foot, these problems improved which seem to confirm the relationship between uneven posture due to the pelvis and lower back misalignments and his discomfort.

His prompt attention to these problems (he is still in his early twenties) may have saved him chronic problems not only in his lower back but also in his left foot and maybe eventually his left knee and/or hip on that side. His response was also faster with fewer visits. If he had have waited it most likely could have become very painful. His problem would have established itself well with strong muscle protection, compensation and taken much longer to respond.

Care Plan:
Doug came three times the first week, once every two weeks and then maintenance of once every six weeks. Doug has subsequently moved out of the area.

Thought to Ponder:

**If deaf people go to court,
is it still a hearing?**

**"One or more vertebrae of the spine
may or may not go out of place very
much. They might give way very
little, and if they do, they are likely
to produce serious complications and
even death, if not properly adjusted."**

Hippocrates, Father of Medicine

3

Connecting with the Past

How the Healing of a Deaf Janitor
Started a Health Care Revolution

It is very helpful to understand the full spectrum of chiropractic by looking at its beginnings – its history. This is an important step in realizing the true miracle of this growing profession primarily founded in the late 1800s, even though there were some primitive forms previous to that time.

Back before the Hippocratic Oath

The first recorded history of healing through manipulation occurred 5000 years ago in Egypt from the great physician Imhotep. He compared the internal workings of our body to the Nile River and pointed out that, "...as a stoppage of the Nile's irrigation system brought disaster to the land, so impingement in the channels of the human system can cause sickness and disease."[6] He made a profound statement, "When you get sick, examine the reason for your sickness and do something about the cause. Health is a matter of correcting the cause."[7] Turtle shell drawings showing spinal adjustments were drawn 4000 years ago in China. Another great physician was born in 470 B.C. in Athens, Greece who became known as the "father of medicine." Hippocrates seemed to "belong to every accredited profession in the healing arts."[8] He figured out that the spine was where many troubles began. He would tie patients to boards and ladders to correct spinal problems. But he didn't develop a system of ideas on how to fix the problems.

Surgeon to the Stadium

Claudius Galen, a Greek, born 130 A.D. in Pergamum located in today's Turkey became the "Surgeon to the Stadium" in that city and later Rome's most renowned medical doctor. He corrected the hand of a noted scholar, Eudemus, by treating the nerves in his neck. This proved quite profound at the time.

Galen was ...

> "the first to correctly describe the spinal column and its articulations, the first experimental neurologist, the first to identify the cranial nerves and the sympathetic nervous system. He made the first experimental cross-sections and vertical sections of the spinal cord, tracing many of the spinal and cranial nerves. He named and defined the cervical, dorsal and lumbar regions, and was among the first to distinguish between those nerves that carry sense impressions to the brain and those that control movement."[9]

Fast Forward

Folk healers in the Dark Ages trampled on sick people's backs. Aulus Celus, a Roman in the first century had compiled a huge encyclopedia which comprised several volumes of general information that had been lost. Eight of these books dedicated to medicine (the fourth book described body parts) were rediscovered in 1426. Because of the invention of the printing press these famous books were published in 1478. Terms named such as vertebrae, humerus, dislocation etc. have remained as standard for over 2000 years. The great anatomist, Andreas Vesalius born in Brussels, Belgium in the early 1500s, dissected cadavers and produced meticulous drawings of the human nervous system with its spine, vertebrae, discs etc. Sir Herbert Barker, born in 1869, became a well-known bonesetter in England. He helped those suffering with damaged joints, particularly knees; he did not, however, recommend surgery. Early in the 19th century physicians did agree that diseases arose in the spine or spinal cord but instead of adjusting the vertebrae in question, they applied leeches and cauteries (hot irons) on these spinal areas.

All through these centuries of learning and discovery, no real organized system of thought relating to the human body such as chiropractic was ever established until D.D. Palmer came along. The emphasis had often been on trying to understand the inner soul and hoping for healing through miracles in various forms of religion rather than through science and reason. The church became very powerful in many lands and often connected itself with hospital care. Doctors' tools were limited. For example, the first microscope wasn't invented until 1590 in the Netherlands. Marcus Bach was an author, researcher of religion and social studies, spokesman at chiropractic conferences, and a friend of B.J. Palmer (D.D. Palmer's son). He traveled the world for several years looking for some prior evidence of chiropractic but his pursuit didn't reveal very much.

Remarkable Chiropractic Beginnings

Daniel David Palmer was born in 1845 in Port Perry, Ontario, Canada (a little town northwest of Toronto). At age 11, his family moved to the U.S. because of his father's grocery business failure. Upon entering adulthood he grew interested in magnetic healing for the body and set up practices first in Burlington, Iowa and later in Davenport, Iowa in 1887. He was always curious about the cause and effect of disease. On September 18, 1895, Dr. Palmer happened to ask the caretaker, Harvey Lillard, in his building how he had become deaf. He was not one of his patients at the time. This gentleman, when he had strained his back 17 years earlier, had heard something "pop" in his back. From then on he complained of hearing problems.

While examining this man's back, Dr. Palmer discovered a bone, called a vertebra, in his spine out of place. Dr. Palmer pushed the vertebra back into place and the caretaker's hearing was improved. He didn't view this as an accidental miracle; with his reasoning ability and previous study he expected the result that happened. This event was the first recorded chiropractic adjustment which caused much excitement and controversy. It challenged the traditional medical concept of creating and maintaining good health. The problem was heightened by enthusiastic believers who made exaggerated claims about what this new approach might achieve. Detractors arose to discredit the methodology and stamp out this profession.

Meanwhile, a Christian clergyman, Rev. Samuel Weed, one of Dr. Palmer's patients, is thought to have put the Greek words for "hand" (cheir) and "done by" (praktoros) together to create the word "chiropractic", meaning "done by the hand."

Passing the Baton

In 1897, Dr. Palmer opened a chiropractic school that graduated 15 people five years later, one graduate being his son Bartlett Joshua (B.J.). B.J. had been 13 years old when his father performed his first chiropractic adjustment and with his very intelligent, confident and fearless nature, he completely understood the significance of his father's discovery even at that young age. Dr. Palmer turned over the administration of the school to B.J. while he finished his last ten years traveling, writing and lecturing in some of the colleges he helped found. He remarked of himself, "The basic principles of chiropractic are not new. They are as old as the vertebrata... I do claim, however ...to create a science which is destined to revolutionize the theory and practice of healing art."[10] "Old Dad Chiro", his affectionate nickname used by many practitioners around the world, died in July, 1913 battling typhoid fever in Los Angeles.

Without B.J.'s involvement, chiropractic would not have survived the early ruthless attempts to discredit its healing ability. He became known as the "Developer" of chiropractic for his desire was to market chiropractic so much that it would become a household word. To do this he started teaching, wrote numerous books on chiropractic and established a radio network that broadcast thousands of hours of his thoughts and data on chiropractic. WOC ("Wonders of Chiropractic"), B.J.'s first radio station, even hired Ronald Reagan (his first sportscasting position). By 1924, one million people were listening daily to the broadcasts. B.J. also later founded one of the first television stations west of the Mississippi.

Knowing the importance of x-rays, B.J. introduced this measuring tool to chiropractic in 1910. Before this the only way a doctor could see inside his patient was to open him up. Surprisingly the x-ray tube had been discovered by Wilhelm Roentgen in 1895 – the same year that his father discovered chiropractic.

Even though B.J. was a most persuasive, charismatic personality, because so many were very skeptical about chiropractic, near the time of his death he retorted in frustration, "They haven't even discovered it now that it is here!"[11] He died in 1961, the president of the Palmer School of Chiropractic from

1906. The baton was then passed along to his son, David D. Palmer (1906-78), who was known as the "Educator" of chiropractic. He assumed the presidency of the school which later became a college.

Highlights of the Time

An article in Psychology Today dated August 24, 2006 called *Immune Boost: This is Spinal Zap* by Katie Gilbert stated this:

> "Chiropractic care was first linked to improved immunity during the deadly flu epidemic of 1917 and 1918. The funny thing was: Chiropractic patients fared better than the general population. This observation spurred a study of the field. The data reported that flu victims under chiropractic care had an estimated .25 percent death rate, a lot less than the normal rate of five percent among flu victims who did not receive chiropractic care."[12]

That is when those in the know finally figured chiropractors just might be on to something! People were dying everywhere. It was awful. But those who went to the chiropractors of the day were 20 times less likely to have died. This story is well documented history. Now that should get the world's attention once more. Swine Flu or the H1N1 Virus appeared on the scene in 1976 and again in 2009 in Mexico when it spread rapidly to the four corners of the globe. Will this pandemic be decreased in size because of the lessons learned during the Spanish flu of 1918? Time will tell when the research is complete. Enhanced immunity in the body was key then and is just as important today.

Chiropractors struggled over proper licensing for numerous years with the result that many were jailed. Herbert Ross Reaver, a graduate of the Palmer School in 1928, was jailed four times in Cincinnati, Ohio. That didn't stop him from giving beneficial chiropractic care to prisoners and guards alike. Licensing came later in various states.

In the 1920s some chiropractors became interested in the effect of chiropractic on mental illness patients. Dr. Gerald Pothoff believed that chiropractic care could better improve psychiatric disorders over regular medical treatment. He opened the first chiropractic hospital, Forest Park Sanitarium, in Davenport, Iowa in 1922. Clear View Sanitarium in Davenport was also established.

Chiropractors readily referred patients to these hospitals. It was just about the time of the great economic depression when families did not have insurance policies and state hospitals were not pleasant places. Dr. W. Heath Quigley, a former director, reported, "The lesson we learned was that beneath the facade of mental illness lives a very human being. Helping to discover that being and releasing him or her has been one of the most thrilling experiences of my life."[13] Dr. Herbert C. Hender, a Palmer faculty member, became a popular lecturer on chiropractic and mental illness.

When soldiers returned from World War II in 1944 many took advantage of government benefits. Thousands enrolled in chiropractic colleges. Today, chiropractic is second only to medicine as the largest primary health care provider in the western world. Approximately 23 chiropractic colleges with over 10,000 students exist worldwide.

The Activator

Since the science of chiropractic began, chiropractors have been using various instruments to make adjustments more comfortable for the patient. In 1901 many were using a "stick method" developed by Thomas H. Storey, a graduate of D.D. Palmer. This was a

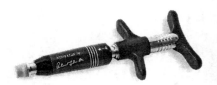

The Activator

wooden mallet and a stick covered with a rubber tip that might have come from a crutch. D.D. Palmer started using a rubber hammer around 1910.

In the 1960s Drs. Warren Lee and Arlan Fuhr modified a "dental impactor, a small instrument designed to force amalgam into cavities in teeth."[14] Unfortunately, this did not produce enough force. Then in 1967 another dentist patient gave these doctors a surgical impact mallet designed to split impacted wisdom teeth. This instrument was modified and became the ancestor to the modern AAI or Activator Adjustment Instrument. When it did not hold up to the demands of a busy chiropractic practice, Freddy Hunziker, a chiropractic student designed and built a more reliable internal mechanism for the Activator. In 1976 the patent was sold to Activator Methods, Inc. and was manufactured by a Swiss-American firm. The AAI remained unchanged until 1994 when the delivery of force was improved through research projects at the University of

Vermont. In 1971 Lee and Fuhr began seminars in Minneapolis to train chiropractors in the use of this instrument and the technique they developed along with it involving leg length measurement to determine body imbalance. These seminars quickly spread to other cities and countries.

A Simple Start

So the start of chiropractic was simple but profound. As with many other professions, the words complicate it. D.D. Palmer figured out that by using his hand to push a bone back to its proper position a man could hear. And the rest is history.

It's Worth the Drive

Name: .... Grant Gallichan
From: .... Newmarket,
Ontario
Treated for: ..... Migraines; Nose
Bleeds; Torn
Knee Ligament;
Childhood
Diseases;
Dizziness

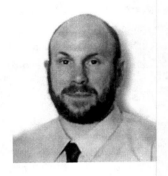

Connection Story

"I am probably one of the first patients that Dr. Côté began treating over 20 years ago when she took over her Erindale Chiropractic Clinic. I had been struggling with migraines and really bad nose bleeds for a very long time. All the medication that I was taking was giving me an ulcer. A friend of mine recommended I go see Dr. Côté. Immediately she asked if I had been in a car accident. I responded that I had been in a big one. This car accident plus my work as an electrician were causing my ailments. I visited her three times a week initially for neck adjustments and it was during the second week that the nose bleeds stopped and the migraines began to subside. Since then our family moved some distance away. But I still travel the distance to her office each month for it is very much worth it to me. My insurance carrier from work, unfortunately, doesn't cover the cost of adjustments. I'm sure if all insurance companies did provide that benefit, medical costs would be cut down significantly.

Whenever I have any injury I make sure Dr. Côté checks me out. Last year I slipped and fell tearing a ligament in my knee. My family doctor recommended surgery but with adjustments from Dr. Côté, ice packs regularly on the knee and exercise to strengthen the surrounding tissue there is no need of surgery.

When my wife, Karen, was pregnant with our second son, Nicholas, we had to take Ethan, our first born to the hospital for tonsillitis. While attending to Ethan, Karen found she couldn't stand up straight. After an adjustment with Dr. Côté she was much better. Dr. Côté told us to bring Ethan in to see her as well. At two years of age, he wasn't eating properly and felt sick all the time. After his neck adjustment his appetite returned and he didn't have a problem with his tonsils after that. As a matter of fact both of our boys have suffered with few or no childhood ailments because we visit Dr. Côté as a family. Ethan was adjusted when he was only three days old and Nicholas two days old as babies. Karen does some lifting at her work and so needs regular treatments.

Over the years I have recommended Dr. Côté's service to others and if the person can't make it to her office because of the distance another chiropractor from the website, www.activator.com, is located. One of my coworkers in particular has suffered with a severely herniated disk in her back but now has received much relief from pain after seeing a chiropractor. With exercises and a nine month process she is much improved.

Dr. Côté is a fabulous person with lots of natural path health care to give as well!"

Comments:

Grant came to my office initially for neck pain and headaches. His exam revealed a deviant neck posture (head jutted forward) along with stiffness in some neck movements. He had suffered from these problems for as long as he could remember. He had suffered from meningitis when he was five plus experienced numerous and memorable falls in his childhood, one of which was falling off a roof when he was only 12. He also endured a "doozy" of a car accident at age 19.

After a month of care he was noticing a decrease in his headaches but also a decrease in his dizziness he had not mentioned initially. With his neck adjustments he gets a lot of relief from the dizziness he took for "granted" – pun intended.

In the past few years Grant rarely has neck pain, headaches or dizziness. We see him and his family regularly for all sort of aches and pain. It's amazing what trouble two young active boys can get themselves into!

Care Plan:

Grant had more frequent visits initially depending on the ailment and then regular monthly treatments for the past twenty years. He has made sure his family members are well cared for also.

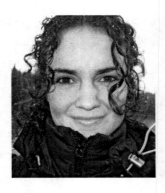

Back on the Plane Again

Name: .... Joanne Pettit-Myers

From: .... North Bay, Ontario

Treated for: ..... Neck Pain; Back Injury; Headaches; Knee Injury; Ulcerative Colitis

"I have been having chiropractic treatments since I was 13 years old. When 4 years old I was hit by a car causing neck and back injuries resulting in headaches. As the headaches persisted, I would only need to have one chiropractic treatment and the headaches would go away. In high school I fell on my knee. At this time I was going to a chiropractor in Hamilton, ON who used the Activator method and upon my next visit he asked me if I had fallen. I had forgotten about this incident but did notice that my knee had become noisy after my fall while running. My knee problem was solved in one visit.

At age 17, I was diagnosed with ulcerative colitis which causes inflammation of the large intestine and blood in the stools. I am now in my 30s and as I have gotten older the inflammation is more constant and can be quite harsh because of the tremendous amount of urgency in going to the washroom. When I moved to Mississauga and upon my mother's recommendation I started visiting Dr. Côté. Her treatments do not relieve all my symptoms but there is a tremendous reduction with regular visits.

Last spring I went to India but unfortunately in my travels I thought I had contracted an antibiotic resistant bacteria (and still may have). I was in the hospital in London, England for two weeks where, although quite nice and eager to help, they couldn't alleviate my symptoms. I came home to Canada seeking medical attention with no luck as well. My preexisting condition of colitis had probably been aggravated by the bacterial organism and therefore I was going to the washroom 40-50 times a day. I lost 30 pounds, was very unhealthy and confined to my house due to washroom demands.

I decided to return to Dr. Côté as it had been about five months since my last visit. My vertebrae directly related to my digestion were much further out of alignment than she had ever seen. I had treatments three

Connection Story

times in the first week and by the Friday I was pretty much back to normal — well, at least normal for me. Weeks and weeks of doctor's visits and medication had little effect but a few trips to the chiropractor and I was on the mend! What I realized after this quick recovery with chiropractic care was that my symptoms had started soon after I was forced into a very difficult yoga position which I now know disturbed my spinal alignment. It turned out that the deranged structure affected the function of the nerves supplying my bowels and gave me symptoms mimicking a bacterial infection.

After two weeks I felt good enough to hop back on the plane to Europe. I am healthier than I've been in years and I am completely off any medication. Although I do believe that my healing process has been helped by a mixture of positive energy and healthy intention, I am grateful to Dr. Côté for starting me back on the path of taking control of my health. I have since then made more dietary changes and mixed with my monthly chiropractic visits, lead almost a symptom free life. I am, as a result, a very outspoken advocate of the benefits of chiropractic treatment."

Comments:

Joanne started her chiropractic journey by seeking help for an annoying knee pain that showed up occasionally when running. Adjustments to her knee and lower back kept her pain free. Later, when faced with a stressful situation her neck would tighten. She would get relief with chiropractic care as is the case with many people.

Upon travelling to India for a yoga retreat she was forced into a very uncomfortable pose. Soon after she developed an acute bout of colitis that left her incapacitated. She went to doctors there who advised her not to travel. She spent a few weeks, still sick, in a foreign country. Losing weight fast and still no better she decided to return home. She had to stop in London as she was too ill to make it all the way home. Again new doctors, new drugs, no better. Upon her return she visited me for a check-up. I found significant problems in her upper lumbar and lower thoracic spine where she felt the discomfort when put in that awkward yoga pose. After only a few adjustments the colitis started to clear. We realized a neurological problem was causing her bowel upset.

Care Plan:

Joanne has had chiropractic care since age 13. At one point after four visits her colitis went away. She is now on a monthly maintenance program.

Connection Story

The Other Side —
The Beginning

Name: .... Doreen Soloduka
From: .... Tiverton, Ontario
Treated for: .... Twisted Spine;
Migraines; Bowel
Problems; Sinus
Problems

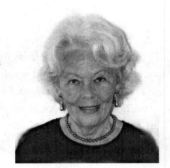

"When I was six, I fell off of a swing. I was taken to the hospital but no bones were found broken. By ten years of age I was beginning to be bothered by back pain and by age twelve I had to crawl up the stairs and come back down on my bottom. I also suffered with bad headaches. I was taken to many doctors whose solutions were only that I had to outgrow my growing pains, just get used to the pain, accept my way of life, or possibly look forward to a body cast or even a wheel chair some day.

As a last resort, my father decided to take me to a chiropractor for pain relief at age fourteen. He had had great success with chiropractic treatments himself; however chiropractic care was not the normal way to proceed in that day. X-rays were taken during my first appointment and revealed that I had a twisted spine. I was like a cork screw. I returned to the chiropractor's office every other day. With my pain gradually decreasing I didn't have to go as often. I became so mobile that by age seventeen I managed to become a cheer leader for our high school football team. I had never been able to do anything like that before and it gave me something to work and strive for.

One Saturday that I was to cheerlead I had an extremely bad headache. My thoughtful boyfriend, Fred, called my chiropractor to arrange a special treatment for me in his office. My headache immediately improved after the adjustment and we were off to the football game. From this incident and others, my boyfriend saw what chiropractic care can do for people. It influenced him to become a chiropractor himself. We married a few years later. He took good care of me as he did with all his chiropractic patients for 40 years until his death. Our two sons, Steve and Stan, also became chiropractors.

I believe I am in better health today than I was as a teenager or even in my 20s or 30s. As a young person, my body was so out of whack and imbalanced. Through the years chiropractic adjustments have helped with my migraine headaches, bowel complaints, sinus problems etc. I visit my son, Stan, every week for a tune up because I can. When he takes my blood pressure and realizes it is up due to some stress in my life, after a treatment it's back down again. I am a living example of what good chiropractic care can do along with healthy nutrition, proper exercise, and a positive attitude about life and me. It was so good that my son, Steve, married Dr. Micheline Côté!"

Comments:

My mother-in-law is an inspiration to anyone watching her. She maintains a schedule that would have any 30 year old spinning. She gardens, urban poles (new sport), does yoga, walks regularly, is super active in her community, does Weight Watchers' counselling, belongs to Toast Masters among other things. Still with all this going on she manages to be there when anyone needs her. When she has a health challenge she strives to solve it with chiropractic care, naturopathy, exercises and diet – without drugs. Now in advanced years she is healthier than most people half her age. Regular chiropractic care I'm sure has a very big part to play in that.

Care Plan:

Doreen has treatments once a week since her son is a chiropractor living close to her.

Thought to Ponder:

When one sits up or sits down, does that mean the same thing?

"Nothing in life is to be feared. It is only to be understood."

Marie Curie

4

Connecting with the Parts

How a Knowledge of Your Body Leads to Improved Long-Term Health

Are you concerned or annoyed over a nagging health problem? A chiropractor is concerned about your nagging symptoms too. But a basic premise of chiropractic science is to address the underlying problem — not just drive the symptoms away. The problem needs to be solved. With every one of my patients I am looking for the root cause of a particular ailment. Understanding our body structure or anatomy and how it works really helps me with that search. So that you can better understand it too you are about to embark upon a "fantastic voyage" into the inner workings of your body, just like the old Sci Fi movie from 1966 called "Fantastic Voyage." (Google "Fantastic Voyage" to see the trailer on this interesting movie.) Don't worry — this is as technical as this book is going to get.

Listen Up Class

First of all, this information is a very condensed version of what we learn at a chiropractic college. As you know the body is extremely complex with all of its various systems and their own special functions. I will only mention the parts that are of particular interest in chiropractic.

Keep in mind that explaining chiropractic to a child will be different than explaining it to a nurse or a doctor untrained in chiropractic. Every person is at a different level of understanding and so the explanation has to be adjusted accordingly. In my office I have to adapt this explanation to the patient I am seeing at the time.

Taking this body tour, you will learn a little embryology (the science of how the body developed before birth), some anatomy (the science of how the body is structured) and some physiology (the science of how the body functions). Armed with that knowledge you will be better able to comprehend how chiropractic works and why it is so good for your health.

Development of the Body before Birth (Embryology)

You might find it amazing that every person evolves from just one tiny cell – a fertilized ovum.

After conception this egg (ovum) that eventually becomes a fully developed human being divides repeatedly for a few weeks until a group of cells called the "morula" is formed. This is the stage when all the cells of the early fetus are just exactly the same or undifferentiated. The cells in the morula haven't yet developed into a particular role in the body.

At this point the nervous system miraculously begins to develop or differentiate itself from some of these cells. That differentiation starts to occur a mere two weeks after conception. This is necessary because the nervous system has to be present to help control the further development of the fetus.

The nervous system is composed of the brain, spinal cord and nerves. It is geographically in the center of the body. Logically it would have to be there first being the core of the body.

The next tissues to differentiate are the skeletal or bony tissues which begin as cartilage. They will develop into bones later to form the frame of the body and the protective tissues around the nervous system.

The skull protects the brain. The spine protects the spinal cord. The heart, lungs, liver, kidneys, stomach, spleen and gall bladder are themselves protected by the rib cage which offers less bony protection than the skull offers the brain.

The brain is completely enclosed by solid bone whereas all the other vital organs are sheltered in a "cage." Have you ever wondered why that is? Obviously the nervous system is important as it is the body's communication system but there is also another reason. The nervous system is particularly vulnerable to damage. Nerve tissue cannot repair itself as all other tissues can. It, therefore, needs to be better protected than any other tissues in the body.

When a nerve is "pinched" in the spine your posture will change and distort to relieve the pressure that causes the irritation on the nerve. We call that change "muscular or postural compensation." Unless you know how to look for it, it is unlikely you will notice it unless it is severe.

Now let's get back to the womb. After the formation of the skeletal tissues, the organs then grow at the end of the nerves like buds on a tree branch in springtime. At the end of the fourth month of development all organs are formed as part of the creation of a perfect little human being.

How is all of this "powered" you may wonder? To describe this power chiropractors use the term "innate intelligence" which just simply means intelligence "born within." This is the energy that is generated in the brain and transmitted by your nerves to every cell of your body. Every muscle moved, every heartbeat initiated, every breath taken, every hormone released, every blood cell produced, every stomach cell replaced is directed by that energy. All body activities are controlled by the force relayed by your nerves. This force keeps your body parts doing the things they are supposed to do in the way they are supposed to do them. Without this power or innate intelligence there is no life.

How the Body Is Structured (Anatomy)

How's the journey thus far? A brief description of how all the body parts are structured will help you better understand how your body works. The body is made of several complex operating systems such as the nervous system, which we have been discussing, the skeletal, circulatory, muscular, reproductive, digestive, hormonal, and immune systems being the main ones. These systems are categorized by the function they perform and are made up of different organs. For instance, the digestive system includes the stomach, liver, gall bladder, pancreas, small and large intestines, just to name a few.

As mentioned previously the nervous system is composed of the brain, the spinal cord and the millions of nerves that connect everything to the brain. The central nervous system is the brain and the spinal cord. These parts are enclosed in the skull and the spine respectively for protection.

The spine consists of four sections. The top section has seven cervical (neck) vertebrae (from the Latin word "vertere" meaning to turn). Did you know that the first bone in the neck (C1) is called the "atlas" from Atlas, the god in mythology who holds the globe of the world? The next section has twelve thoracic (chest) vertebrae where the 24 ribs are attached plus five lumbar (lower back) vertebrae. These three sections allow the trunk of the body to move and flex. Below the fifth lumbar, the sacrum and the coccyx are found, commonly known as the tailbone. These bottom vertebrae are fused and practically immobile.

A cushion named a vertebral disk separates and unites each vertebrae. This cushion acts much like a shock absorber and allows for an opening between two adjacent vertebrae. Out of these openings, called the "intervertebral foramina", a pair of nerves exit, one on each side. These spinal nerves supply all of the different tissues or organs in the body.

The Nervous System

The nervous system is divided into two components – the voluntary and the autonomic. You might want to call them the "conscious" nervous system and the "automatic" nervous system. The voluntary nervous system, as the word suggests, is under conscious or thinking control. When you want to move your arm, you think it and your nervous system communicates it to your arm muscles via your nerves and it happens. The mental impulse is generated in the brain and the message is transmitted by chemical and electrical forces to the arm and back again to the brain. It is mind boggling to reflect on how many of those messages travel back and forth to allow you to do all that you have to do moment by moment. Also consider what would happen if these message pathways were obstructed. It would be as if there is a lot of static on your phone line or an irritating echo that makes it hard to communicate with the other person. This definitely causes a problem.

The autonomic, on the other hand, performs without conscious or with non-thinking effort from you and controls functions such as heart rate, digestive actions, release of hormones and the like. There is no thinking necessary on your part while these millions of messages are traveling along the nerve pathways doing their job.

Furthermore, the autonomic nervous system is itself divided into two parts: the sympathetic and the parasympathetic. The sympathetic nervous system takes care of your regular unconscious functions when you are in a situation of stress. When the sympathetic nervous system kicks in, for example, blood flow is transferred from your digestion to your muscles so that you are ready to run away from or fight the situation that is stressing you. Your pupils dilate so you can see better, your hearing is heightened, your breathing increases and so does your heart rate just to name a few things. As well, all digestive and other regular functions unnecessary for fight or flight are put on hold for the time of stress. This increases the blood supply available to your muscles and heart.

The parasympathetic nervous system, on the other hand, controls the same body functions as the sympathetic nervous system but when circumstances are normal and not in a state of stress. The blood flow is directed to your digestive tract away from your muscles. The heart rate stays at its normal resting rate since it does not need to pump more blood to more muscles. Breathing is at its regular frequency and healing functions are heightened.

Imagine

Just imagine, as an illustration, a hospital setting with its personnel taking care of the various needs of their patients. All of a sudden the hospital is under attack because it is in a war zone or encounters an emergency such as an earthquake or hurricane. Personnel quickly change their focus from care to keeping their patients safe. They move them away from the windows or transfer them to a more secure place in the basement. Food preparation and distribution are delayed until the crisis has passed. Elective surgery is no longer scheduled for the duration of the emergency. Similarly and incredibly your body functions much like this. The parasympathetic nervous system controls things when it is business as usual. When there is stress or a crisis the sympathetic nervous system takes over. All these changes occur without you having to make one single decision. Therein lies the importance of a well functioning and freely communicating nervous system.

How the Body Functions (Physiology)

The nervous system is your body's communication system. It would be quite lengthy and complex to describe the millions of nerve pathways and connections and how the chemistry of transmitting messages works. It is also beyond the scope of this book to do so. What is worthwhile knowing though is that the communicating done through the nervous system can be either conscious or unconscious as previously mentioned.

The unconscious or autonomic control takes care of many important activities and regulates them every second. The heart rate for example is changed if you go from sitting in the theater to walking outside to go home.

These adjustments to the heart rate are done without any decision on your part and occur based on many indicators or sensors within your body. Your brain, also, has to know what is going on around you to make the appropriate adjustments to its systems, so it is equipped with a selection of different sensory organs that perceive touch, light or deep pressure, body position, pain, temperature, sight, hearing and smell.

All these sensors send messages to the brain constantly so that the body can regulate itself all the time. A loop of incoming messages is formed influencing the outgoing messages. This loop has been affectionately termed the "safety pin cycle" by early chiropractors because it illustrates normal or disrupted nerve pathways whether the pin is open or closed. It is open when there is a subluxation and closed when the nervous system is allowing messages to travel to and from.

It is much easier to understand the nerve disruption in the voluntary nervous system as it is felt on a conscious level. In your brain you think you want to move your arm and the message is sent to the arm muscles to do just that. But in order to move it properly the brain has to understand the arm's present position so it can move the appropriate muscles to cause that change. Again if there is interference in the nerves along the "safety pin", the sensors are not able to give the appropriate data to the brain and the ensuing action will be less effective. The muscle might be weak or the movement shaky or inappropriate.

It is a bit more difficult to grasp what happens when your autonomic nervous system is interfered with by a misalignment or subluxation. With all the sensory input your brain needs to regulate itself, even the most basic functions can be decreased or increased when receiving inappropriate or incomplete information. Your brain, in turn, takes inappropriate actions. That is why people sometimes have cold feet in a warm bed, a fast heart rate without running, or more acid in the stomach without eating a meal. Chaos occurs then in the regulation of the most basic functions because the proper functioning of the nervous system is disturbed.

So how are these messages transmitted in your body? The power is electrical in nature. This force can be measured with an electrocardiogram or electroen-cephalogram test, commonly known as an ECG and EEG. In recent years chiropractors have been using surface electromyography or EMG to measure the electrical activity in the muscles along the spine. The information we get from this is very useful. Electrical activity can easily be measured on either side of the spine and uneven results indicate uneven electrical output at that spinal level which will reveal a subluxation or disruption in that nerve output.

As you can see your nervous system is of vital importance to you and a well aligned spine is necessary for it to function well. The chiropractor's job is to make sure that your structure is as well aligned as possible so that your nervous system is functioning at its full potential without interferences. As Thomas Edison said so well, "The doctor of the future will give no medicine but will interest himself and his patients in the 'care of the human frame', in diet and in the cause and prevention of disease."

Simple Truths

So did you learn something new from this "fantastic voyage"? It really is all summed up by the following few principles:
1. The body is a self-healing and self-regulating organism.
2. A well functioning nervous system is essential for proper healing and self-regulation.
3. A misalignment or subluxation interferes with the proper functioning of the nervous system; therefore it interferes with great health.
4. Chiropractors are the only health professionals trained to detect and correct these interferences or subluxations.
5. When subluxations are corrected the body functions better and most symptoms, including pain, can then subside.

Connection Story

Hands Up Everyone

Name: .... Sue T.
From: .... Aurora, Ontario
Treated for: ..... Lower Back Pain; Foot Injury;
Dislocated Knee

"I love all kinds of sports and so it is not surprising for you to learn that I graduated from physical education at university. Unfortunately, several years ago I began having pain in the right side of my lower back. The pain would become so debilitating that it was difficult for me to function and even walk. My family doctor prescribed heavy duty drugs to decrease the inflammation and pain. I did all the stretching exercises I could to strengthen my muscles and help my back return to proper fitness. The pain would last for days and I would continue to pop pills — something I really didn't like doing. My back would go out over the simplest thing such as stepping off of a curb. I could hardly walk, bend over or sit down.

My friend who was also in physical education had been in a similar situation, often being stuck in bed with her pain. When she started getting better through Dr. Côté's treatments I became interested. I was really inspired to make an appointment as I was planning a three week trip to Europe. I really wanted to travel but was very fearful that I would have trouble with my back on this trip.

After my consultation and adjustment with Dr. Côté I proved to be fine, thankfully. I continued seeing Dr. Côté but we just couldn't narrow down the cause of my problem that would set off the pain. Then one day she asked me if I could remember putting my hands above my head for any particular action. That was it! I was an avid camper for 20 years taking children on canoe trips as a canoe instructor. That meant hauling and holding 12 canoes separately over my head as we portaged. She identified my weakness of lifting and holding something over my head which action I must be careful to avoid forever.

Seven years ago I unexpectedly stepped in a pothole which tore the ligaments in the arch of my foot. The doctor put me on pain killers and then I immediately went to Dr. Côté's office. Every other day she taped my foot after each adjustment to keep it in place. This really helped it to heal and I didn't miss one day of work.

Last February there was another incident at school and I was injured. My knee was partially dislocated. I couldn't walk and had to go on crutches. More powerful pain killers this time! Dr. Côté was able to put my knee back in place and I was able to walk. I did have to have surgery eventually but it was minor in comparison to what the doctor was predicting. My knee is growing stronger today. I owe a great deal of gratitude to Dr. Côté for she never gave up on me. She even learned a new chiropractic technique to help my leg relax and get the most out of the adjustment.

I have recommended her services to other teachers in both of my schools where I have worked. My mother at age 76 was not able to use her elbows while caring for her grandchildren. She always has been healthy with naturopathic methods. Even the physiotherapist she went to couldn't figure out her problem. Dr. Côté gave her an adjustment from her shoulders to her fingers and after two weeks, this really made a difference in the quality of her life.

Dr. Côté always shows a spirit of helpfulness and determination no matter the crisis."

Comments:

Sue has been a patient in my office for many years. I have seen her for a variety of problems as she has been hard on her body being an enthusiastic physical education teacher.

Many of her physical conditions have responded well to chiropractic care, so it is always what she tries first when dealing with a health problem whether it is a back problem, her bad knee that was injured many years ago, her foot, shoulder or neck.

She has saved herself taking many bottles of pain killers I'm sure through the years which is always better for your health.

Sue lives the chiropractic lifestyle and has referred many of her colleagues, friends and family for care as she sees first hand the benefit of such a lifestyle.

Care Plan:

Sue initially had eight visits and now is on a once a month maintenance program or we see her for more visits if a new concern arises.

Connection Story

Surgery or Chiropractic Care?

Name: .... Gloria W.
From: .... Acton, Ontario
Treated for: ..... Carpal Tunnel
Syndrome; Lower
Back Pain

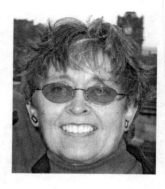

"I began experiencing pain in my right wrist in the late 1990s. My job involved a lot of computer work. Upon contacting my physician I learned that I had Carpal Tunnel Syndrome. My doctor suggested I purchase a brace and wear it. No pain killers were prescribed. I learned that my neighbor suffered with the same problem and had gone through surgery to alleviate the pain. I certainly didn't want to go that route!

My friend recommended contacting Dr. Côté which I did. The first visit for consultation included an x-ray. She examined my whole body and found out that I actually needed an adjustment in my neck as it wasn't aligned properly. I needed two visits each week for six weeks and then once a month regularly for maintenance to keep this problem from reoccurring. Fortunately my insurance plan covered all expenses.

I once put my back out and could hardly move. Another friend suggested I go straight to see Dr. Côté! She soon had me right after a couple of visits. I have had no further pain since and gladly refer others.

My husband and I moved to another community and now have found a chiropractor here who does know of Dr. Côté.

When my husband, John, saw my improvement along with encouragement from a friend, he decided to make an appointment for himself. He had been to another chiropractor previously but was not impressed. However, I will let him tell his story."

Comments:

Gloria first came to see me because of her right hand pain. Her exam and x-rays showed that her cervical (upper) spine was also in trouble showing deviations and disc degeneration. Adjusting both her hand and neck gave Gloria quick relief. In six visits she was 70% and after one more week her problem was completely gone. Gloria has had a hand numbness problem through the years associated with the same structural weakness in her neck but because of traveling and living out of the province off and on, we were not able to prevent it completely. Every time she was in town, though, she was adjusted and felt better quickly.

Care Plan:
Gloria required 12 visits and then came to see me once a month thereafter until she moved to another town.

Get Activated!

Name: .... John W.
From: .... Acton, Ontario
Treated for: ..... Lower Back Pain

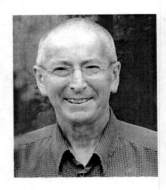

"My first encounter with a chiropractor was after I slipped and fell while crossing a stream. Not only did I suffer impact injury, but in attempting to recover my balance had twisted my lower back. The chiropractor used traditional manipulation over a series of treatments with no marked improvement. In fact, some days I felt worse rather than better and I began to doubt the effectiveness of the hit and miss adjustments. Following one session I felt much worse and became almost incapacitated with pain. One further adjustment restored the status quo; I was no better than I had been when I started, and I concluded that chiropractic was an inexact science and therefore decided not to go back for any further treatments.

However, a friend recommended Dr. Côté because she uses the Activator method, and persuaded me to at least give her a try. At that time, I was unable to stand erect for more than a few minutes before feeling intense pain and discomfort in my lower back, and also numbness in my right thigh and pain in my left knee when walking. After examining me and studying the x-ray of my spine, Dr. Côté informed me she could give me some relief, but suspected the problem with my knee would need other medical attention. Nevertheless, after only a few adjustments using the Activator, I noticed marked and steady improvement until all the pain and discomfort was gone.

I have confidence in Dr. Côté and in the chiropractic method she employs, using the Activator."

Comments:

John had right sacroiliac and hip pain when he first came to my office. He had broken his toe when he was young and feels it affected the way he walked even that far back. His knee, also on the right side, was occasionally bothersome.

He was adjusted for a few weeks to realign his pelvis, hips and knee and then given exercises to mobilize one of his lower back discs. He responded well to this type of care as one month later he was pain free and exercising regularly.

Then because of extensive traveling we could not adjust him for long periods of time. I would see him occasionally while he was in town to straighten out what plane rides, different beds, and carrying luggage managed to misalign.

John and Gloria have moved to another town. Since seeing the value of chiropractic they are now making appointments with another chiropractor closer to home.

Care Plan:

John only needed a few visits — three times a week for a few weeks — before he was feeling fine.

Thought to Ponder:

How can fat chance and slim chance mean the same thing?

"The greatest discovery of any generation is that human beings can alter their lives by altering their attitudes of mind."

Albert Schweitzer

Connecting with a Plan

How One Small Step Will Dramatically Improve Your Health

When you hurt yourself or something goes wrong with your health, your nervous system immediately starts working to find a solution to repair the problem. You are obviously not aware of the millions of actions that take place to deal with these troubles; however if you could take a closer look you would be amazed at the marvelous ways your body innately tries to heal itself.

Your Body's Healing Strategies

When you accidentally cut the skin on your hand, bleeding occurs first of all. One of the functions of bleeding is to help wash away impurities. Redness with a bit of swelling around the cut will then appear. You will also feel pain and might even experience heat around the wound. The response to trauma, such as in this injury example, is called the inflammatory process.

Through this process your body brings fluids carrying white blood cells and other types of cells to the damaged spot both to repair and prevent infection. Pain will discourage you to hit or scratch the wound again therefore protecting it from further damage. The heat enhances the ability of the white blood cells to more readily kill the nasty invaders that can cause infections. At this stage getting rid of these activities with pain killers or anti-inflammatories would be counterproductive. A better objective would be to enhance the flow of messages between the brain and the rest of your body. This would allow the body to perform to its full potential and heal the cut appropriately.

After a few hours a scab forms over the wound. This remarkable process protects and allows the skin underneath to heal. All of this happens on its own under the direction of your autonomic nervous system. You know that if you scratched that scab off too early it would lead to more bleeding and lengthen the healing time for the injury.

Similarly injured tendons or ligaments, after the initial inflammatory process, develop scar tissue. This tissue heals and repairs any tears and bruising. It is not a mistake in your body that should be reversed. You need to be patient and allow this scar tissue to do its job. In time when enough of the damage in the ligament or tendon has been fixed, the scar tissue will dissolve and gradually disappear on its own if the cause of the damage has been addressed. It is plain to see that doing a lot of stretching of the ligament or tendon being repaired before enough healing has taken place is also counterproductive.

Changes for Coping

Another way that your body deals with an injury is through muscular changes such as muscle spasms or postural adaptations. Have you ever seen the posture of someone with bad sciatica? The person is not straight, often bending to one side or leaning forward. A wry neck (or torticollis) is a similar condition. The neck seems stuck in an unusual position. This awkward pose occurs to prevent nerves from being "pinched" or disturbed any further. If you look closely at yourself in the mirror you might observe more subtle muscular compensations such as uneven ears, shoulders, or hip levels. Look at the bottom of your shoes. Do you notice uneven wear? These are all possible signs of postural adaptations to a problem.

Also, there are numerous, natural chemical changes that occur with pain to help repair an injury. Some chemicals and cells fight infections, some decrease pain, while others develop or lessen the inflammatory process. All these actions are under the control of the nervous system. They do their job spontaneously without any outside help or conscious effort on your part.

If something interferes with the nervous system then all these activities are not as well controlled. From postural adaptations to the delivery of appropriate chemicals to the right amount of muscle tension, all will happen with a little less organization, ease and effectiveness; therefore increasing the time for healing of the injury.

If symptoms are persistent it could mean that your body can no longer deal with the problem by its compensations because your nervous system is interfered with and cannot cope appropriately. It has become overwhelmed. How, then, are you going to handle this situation? It is time for action.

False Solution #1: Ignore

One solution people frequently try is to ignore the trouble. For instance, you may have experienced walking with a pebble in your shoe. It is bearable at first but if you continue to ignore this irritating intruder it will definitely get on your nerves.

"But it's not life threatening," you remark under your breath. And so you keep on walking with the pebble in your shoe even though it is getting very uncomfortable. You then notice that you have worn a hole in your sock. With its constant rubbing on the skin of your foot a bleeding sore may occur that can lead to infection and even more pain and aggravation in the long run. Eventually you start limping to avoid the pain and bring on new problems caused by walking unevenly.

When you finally decide to deal with the cause of the problem and untie your shoe to remove the pebble, you wonder why you have waited so long before getting rid of the annoyance. Do you remember the feeling of relief you experienced when walking again without the pebble in your shoe? A comparable feeling occurs when you get to the cause of a lingering problem solved successfully with chiropractic care. It is a frequent occurrence in a chiropractor's office.

False Solution #2: Desensitize

Another popular method in coping with pain is to numb it with pain killers or artificially reduce the inflammation with medication. Many people know that a fever has a role in fighting a virus or bacteria, but fewer are aware that inflammation also plays an important part in healing tissues that have been injured. Inflammation is not a problem in itself; it is an integral part of your healing system.

When taking pain killers a problem can become worse. You may not be fully aware that you need to protect the injured area during regular daily activities.

That is the purpose of pain! When you take a drug, you have numbed your body's signal of protection. This can be counterproductive to your healing process; further damage and pain can occur. Anti-inflammatories are generally successful at decreasing inflammation but have they really resolved the fundamental cause for the trouble in the first place? Some experts say that if you have to take the medication for more than a week, there is an underlying problem causing the inflammation to continue and this cause obviously needs to be corrected.

False Solution #3: Avoid

A third solution often used to deal with a health issue is to avoid doing what makes the condition worse. For example, if your digestive system is not functioning at its best, you might have trouble digesting onions. Most people can digest them, so why can't you? It is not the onions themselves that cause the problem but the inability of your digestive tract to process the onions. So how do you cope with that? You tend to avoid them by pushing them to the side of your plate or by not eating foods cooked with onions — not life threatening you could say, but much less flavorful.

Similarly, if you have a joint that hurts or an ache in your back when you bend to the left, instead of having the mechanical difficulty corrected, you tend to avoid doing the movements that hurt too much. In my opinion, this is the most depressing way to handle a health problem. The less you move, the stiffer your body gets and the less you will tend to do. Gradually over time, you may find yourself avoiding more and more activities. Eventually you might even lose the ability to do all the things you love.

False Solution #4: Self-Doctor

People can become quite ingenious or resourceful when they don't want to make an appointment with a health care professional. A 95-year old father of one of my patients tried to carve a wooden tooth to fill in the gaping hole where he had lost a tooth in the side of his mouth just because he didn't want to go to the dentist. As you might guess it really didn't work.

Do you ever think you can solve a problem yourself? For example, you might crack your joint with applying a force to it in many directions. You may achieve a popping sound if you bend your finger forwards, backwards or sideways but does that correct the misalignment? Probably not, as the force applied isn't specific to the problem. In order to accomplish a chiropractic adjustment, the force used has to be directed so it can reduce the subluxation if it exists. Then and only then can it be called a chiropractic adjustment.

The True Solution

The appropriate course of action when you have a health concern is obviously not listed above. You must deal with the "pebble in your shoe" – the cause of the malfunction, inflammation or pain. Your chiropractor is trained to detect, analyze and correct misalignments or subluxations in your spine and joints so that you can return to your normal active life again.

Even if you are not certain that your particular symptom can be helped with chiropractic care, it may be worthwhile to set aside your previous beliefs about this growing science and schedule an exam with a chiropractor to determine if you have structural problems that should be addressed. Most patients telling their stories in this book may have had similar reservations initially. Where would they be today if they hadn't given chiropractic a try? It ended up being the true solution that they were seeking.

Think Outside the Box

When you consider these factors, your view is expanded about the various health issues that chiropractic care helps to address. Don't limit your quest for better health to just improvement from aches and pain. Think enhanced function as well because if you can get relief from the pain of a pinched nerve, you can also get relief from the malfunction effect of a pinched nerve.

I am frequently asked about certain difficult conditions such as migraines, fibromyalgia, chronic fatigue syndrome, lupus etc. Many wouldn't consult a chiropractor for these ailments but I have seen my share of patients who have experienced improvement from challenging health situations like these.

In over 25 years of practice, the majority of my patients suffering with migraines have responded favorably. I remember less than five patients I had to refer out to another health care specialist after a month or two of care.

I have also had a few success stories of patients diagnosed with fibromyalgia when there wasn't excessive toxicity or stress associated with these cases. It is more difficult to measure the percentage of response as these sufferers are less common in chiropractors' offices than victims with lower back pain. They are frequently told that nothing can help their situation.

Such diseases as chronic fatigue syndrome and lupus are even less commonly seen in my office and are not well understood by any health professional. These problems, though, result from a weakened immune system. A few studies have shown that chiropractic adjustments have very positive effects on the immune system and could therefore be helpful with such conditions. If these patients are subluxated their chances of improvement would be greater.

A recent study has also shown that chiropractic adjustments of the spine have some brain function effects as measured by EEG. These effects show dramatic improvement in brain function comparing before and after cervical spinal manipulation. With these results in mind you can see the potential of chiropractic adjustments on your health beyond the resolution of aches and pain. It is through these brain and immune system effects that chiropractic could benefit these difficult conditions.

If I had a member of my family stricken with any of these ailments, I would plan to put chiropractic care at the top of my list of recommendations. If your nervous system is irritated in one way or another, you may experience some of the following consequences: you cannot sleep well at night; you cannot properly process food; the food is less easily absorbed; you may have difficulty in eliminating waste; you cannot exercise with ease; you cannot cope with stress appropriately; and you may even have a hard time getting pregnant. These functions are very basic for you and vital to your well being. The healthier "you" comes with a well functioning nervous system.

Taking Control

Certainly, when you have a fall or an accident it is important for the chiropractor to check things out. You don't always know if your structure has been misaligned or disturbed as you often don't see it with an untrained eye. Most times you might not even feel it at first. Vertebrae might have shifted and you may not experience the pain for several days, weeks or even months until tissues get too irritated or you are unable to compensate enough to alleviate the symptoms. It is too bad we cannot see what is going on inside our own bodies.

So who is to know? Your chiropractor of course! The job of this professional is to detect and correct vertebral misalignments or subluxations; then good things happen. The nervous system is able to function more normally; joints move more freely with less pain. The body can better use its natural built-in functions to do the greatest amount of healing possible on its own. A chiropractor adjusts misalignments in the spine so that the nervous system can better attempt to heal what needs to be helped or fixed.

If your greatest desire is to be free of your particular health problem, then you need to put a plan in place. You have to take control of your condition and try the available avenues that are the most natural, least invasive and most beneficial for your body. What if there is real hope in chiropractic care? What if you don't give it a try and sadly miss out on years of vastly improved health?

A Warning About Exercise

Here is one last thought in the long list of benefits from a chiropractic evaluation. Consider how vital regular exercise has become in the public consciousness. Exercise, indeed, helps maintain a healthy body but if your spine or other joints are poorly aligned, then exercise can cause problems because it makes you more susceptible to joint or muscle injury. You have heard it said that you should not start a rigorous exercise program before you consult with your doctor. It is equally true that you should start regular monitoring by your chiropractor to assure you will do more good than harm when you start exercising.

This kind of preventative thinking and planning is particularly important if you want to embark on a new sport or a new type of exercise as I have often seen many problems arise when people change their routine of physical activities. With any workout you will consistently feel better if your body is properly aligned. You will have a better range of motion so that you can conduct your new or old exercise regime effectively and safely. This will allow better strength gain and performance in the long run; just ask athletes like Lance Armstrong, Dan O'Brien, Tiger Woods, and Arnold Schwarzenegger.

Other Considerations

My purpose in providing this information is obviously to help everyone achieve greater health with less pain and suffering. There are also other reasons to consider such as financial and environmental advantages. The cost of medical care has soared in recent years and does not always bring great results. I think with a health care paradigm shift towards more natural and less invasive health care, billions of dollars could be saved. (Additional information coming on this topic in Chapter 7.)

The environmental reasons for using natural approaches to health are very understandable. The more drugs people take, the more our environment, water and soil become polluted with the excretions of these substances. The experts are now able to measure the by-products of medications in our water and we must be careful not to overwhelm the delicate balance of nature. So your decision not to act and take care of your health in a more natural way can have an impact not just on you, but also on the people around you, the economy and the environment.

Waiting Room Anticipation

You have finally decided to try chiropractic care. On your first visit you might feel a little apprehensive as you would with any new experience but after a short wait, you meet the chiropractor and start to get acquainted. Your worries dissolve and work can then start on your quest for better health. The more relaxed you are the easier the chiropractor can care for you. Remember to bring pleasant, positive thoughts along with you.

Be open-minded, accept recommendations given and follow through on them. It takes time to correct problems that have been long in duration. Be patient and cooperate as much as possible. Be assured you and your chiropractor have the same goal in mind – your improved health.

As you leave the office after your initial treatment you may have to admit you feel just a little better, or at least different. Your plan has been put into action. You may notice some relief of stress and even find hope for the future. You detect a smile forming on your face as you savor the moment.

In a few weeks you are probably going to start feeling like a new person with added bounce in your step. If a friend referred you to their chiropractor, why not take that person out to dinner to celebrate the fact that they helped you find a new plan? And why not refer others as your friend has done for you? You'll want everyone you love to gain higher levels of health just as you have realized.

Connection Story

Way Back When

Name:	Raymond Froh
From:	Mississauga, Ontario
Treated for:	Lower Back Pain; Upper Back Pain; Numbness in Arm

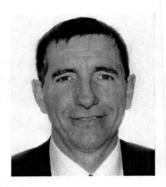

"My story is amazing! I was roller blading with my son a couple of years ago and wrenched my lower back. From that day forward I would start each Monday suffering with pain and by the Friday of each week I could hardly stand up. This continued for about a year until one morning I got up and found myself listing ten degrees to one side. I knew I had to do something as the Aspirin bottle was not helping enough. My father-in-law had gone through the same problem 6 months previously and had been fixed up by Dr. Côté. I finally made an appointment with Dr. Côté myself and learned from her preliminary check-up that she could quite easily help with the lower back problem; however my upper back problem was the real issue.

Nineteen years previous to my visit with Dr. Côté, I had hurt my upper back by putting a telephone-pole-sized pole into the ground while helping to build a "pole" barn out in Saskatchewan. I had learned to live with the pain but always had to be cautious regarding my activities. No rough housing with my kids allowed. When I bumped my head going into the shower, ouch did it hurt! The fear of the onset of debilitating pain was always there. I did go to my family doctor who prescribed muscle relaxants. I would consume hundreds of Aspirins.

Dr. Côté was able to help my lower back problem very quickly; but the progress with my upper back was very slow. It took over a year, starting with three visits a week for several weeks and then that program was reduced to once a week. Today my Aspirin quota is down to six tablets a year for an occasional headache. If I get hurt doing a particular activity, it is wonderful because I know the pain will go away. My body is in better shape and I am able to do activities I haven't done in years due to Dr. Côté's excellent chiropractic care. Currently, I am again off work with another lower back injury because I now feel so full of life that I perform tasks and activities that are not really age appropriate!

I am so grateful to Dr. Côté for the quality of life I now have and would have gladly paid thousands of dollars in exchange for my present health. I see her once a month for check-ups or for the unexpected injury that does arise. My whole life has been changed because I can do the activities I want to be engaged in and am able to exercise better.

My wife, Kathryn, was feeling numbness in her arm a couple of years ago. She went to the hospital several times to make sure she wasn't having a stroke but nothing was found. That was very disconcerting. After visiting Dr. Côté's office a few times it is a non-issue today. Something must have been out of alignment that has been corrected.

Since our very positive experiences in our family, we have recommended Dr. Côté's service to several people also struggling with health issues. Many of them have made appointments and have seen good results. We will definitely continue to be this chiropractor's lifelong advocate."

Comments:
Ray has been coming to my office for chiropractic care for many years and we have dealt with lower back injuries and neck injuries with him when he has had falls or lifted docks at his cottage in the spring or the like.

His main comment, though, when he comes in for his monthly visits is that he can do so much more than he used to do. He has more energy and feels more "solid" as he has tried to describe this to me. Sometimes it is not just the pain that matters for people but rather function and how active they can remain.

It seems that way for Ray as he is thrilled to be able to get all his work done without compromising his health and feeling unwell.

Care Plan:
Raymond came three times a week for several weeks, then decreasing his visits to once a month when he feels well.

Connection Story

Can You Hear Me Now?

Name: .... Robert Regular
From: .... Mississauga, Ontario
Treated for: .... Arm Pain; Shoulder Pain; Hip Pain;
          Foot Pain; Ear Noise

"When I first came to Dr. Côté's clinic I was having a great deal of pain in my right arm and shoulder. I had visited my family doctor and after x-rays he suggested neck exercises to help relieve the pain. If that failed eventual surgery would be needed.

My son and his family are patients of Dr. Côté whom they recommended saying, 'She will be honest and if she feels she cannot help you, she will say so.'

I secured an appointment, was assessed, and after a few short visits, I was able to move my arm with increased strength and less pain. I was not really surprised at the effectiveness of chiropractic care as I have known people who have experienced remarkable results. What did surprise me was how quickly the treatment produced results. My body strengthened considerably and now I feel so much better being able to work without pain. I have more energy and rebound quickly from any setback.

Perhaps the most astonishing reaction to chiropractic treatment has been the relief of ear noise (hissing and tone sounds) that had plagued me for five years. I was informed by previous physicians that this noise was industry related and that I would have to live with it. Also since starting chiropractic care, I can now walk easier. I had experienced hip and foot pain before. I don't need pain killers any more. I continue to visit Dr. Côté's office for maintenance. I only make it two or three times a year as part of each year I reside in Newfoundland.

This all has been so good for me that I inform my coworkers and family how productive it is. My uncle who is a senior citizen in Newfoundland has visited a chiropractor there and a long time back problem has nearly disappeared.

Thank you Dr. Côté for your care and encouragement!"

Comments:

When I met Robert the first time, he had severe right shoulder and neck pain. He continued at the age of 57 to work hard labor jobs full time. In addition, he had suffered an injury when an elevator clipped his right shoulder causing increasing pain.

It has been amazing to see him respond despite the hard work, injuries, car accidents, and more hard work. The last two years have been almost pain free for Robert and now at age 68 he is still continuing to work as hard as before.

It is also interesting that Robert had contended with annoying ear ringing for a long time which was helped significantly with his adjustments. He had not mentioned this to me initially but as it started to subside we realized that the noise was lessening with his chiropractic care.

In Robert's case we supplemented his care with exercises for his posture and shoulders to enhance improvement. His almost frozen shoulder responded miraculously to chiropractic adjustments and these exercises.

Care Plan:

Robert came for a few visits and now sees me only two or three times a year when he is in the province. He saw me three times a week for eight weeks at the beginning. When he has had subsequent problems he responds in two to three weeks usually.

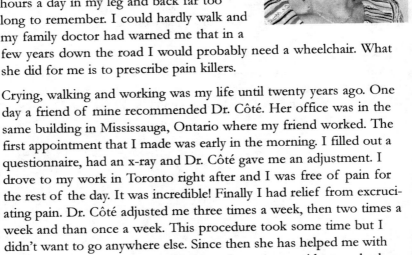

Crying, Walking and Working

Name: .... Ana Bracko
From: .... Mississauga, Ontario
Treated for: .... Sciatica; Migraines; Stress; Neck Pain

"I had been suffering with sciatic pain 24 hours a day in my leg and back far too long to remember. I could hardly walk and my family doctor had warned me that in a few years down the road I would probably need a wheelchair. What she did for me is to prescribe pain killers.

Crying, walking and working was my life until twenty years ago. One day a friend of mine recommended Dr. Côté. Her office was in the same building in Mississauga, Ontario where my friend worked. The first appointment that I made was early in the morning. I filled out a questionnaire, had an x-ray and Dr. Côté gave me an adjustment. I drove to my work in Toronto right after and I was free of pain for the rest of the day. It was incredible! Finally I had relief from excruciating pain. Dr. Côté adjusted me three times a week, then two times a week and than once a week. This procedure took some time but I didn't want to go anywhere else. Since then she has helped me with migraine headaches, stress, neck injury from a car accident, and other problems throughout the years. My visits to Dr. Côté are now every two months for check-ups. She is always there to help me with any concerns I may have.

Chiropractor adjustments are lasting and painless. I found that regular maintenance with this type of care will help you keep your body in good health. Dr. Côté has given me back my health and my life. I recommend her service to everyone."

Comments:

Many years ago Ana suffered from terrible leg pain diagnosed as sciatica. Her right leg was the worst. She responded initially quite quickly to chiropractic care and was able to decrease her check-ups to once a month before too long. I gave her exercises to help a degenerating disc in her lower back.

Ana is the kind of patient that follows instructions to the letter. We can safely say that her lifestyle now is very active, even with a car accident in

Connection Story

the package which occurred about 15 years ago. She is pain-free and drug-free! She schedules visits to our office every two months now to get checked and has very few complaints to report.

Care Plan:
Ana had office visits three times a week for a few weeks, then we gradually decreased the frequency of her visits to now once every two months.

Connection Story

Listening to a Friend

Name: .... Viviene Whittle-Smith

From: .... Brampton, Ontario

Treated For: .... Shoulder Pain; Hip Pain; Right Hand Pain; Back Pain

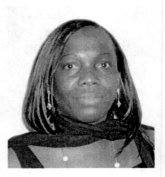

"A bone had slipped out in my shoulder. I had been suffering with pain from it for about two months. I visited my medical doctor three times but even with an x-ray the problem couldn't be found. My doctor prescribed pain killers but the pain kept recurring.

My co-worker referred me to Dr. Côté and after one treatment on a Wednesday I felt better on Thursday, the very next day. I saw her for the next two weeks and since then the pain has not returned. Soon after, I experienced pain in my hip. Again going to my family doctor I found out through an x-ray that I have the beginnings of osteoarthritis. I returned to Dr. Côté's office for another two weeks of treatment and now I only have to schedule an appointment every two months to get checked.

One morning I woke up experiencing pain in my right hand so I immediately made an emergency call to Dr. Côté's office and was able to get right in for treatment. I now know to call her office first for help. This has been a learning experience for me as I didn't realize before that chiropractic can relieve pain other than in the back. And what I really like is I don't have to sit in the waiting-room as long as I do for my family doctor!

My husband, Orville, who is very hard to convince, saw the quick difference in me and so he decided to see Dr. Côté for his back pain. About five years ago he had lifted something incorrectly. Ever since, particularly when gardening or doing some other strenuous activity, the pain reoccurs. He had gone for medical advice but all that was prescribed were exercises with no pain killer. After three treatments in the chiropractor's office he is now also on a two-month check-up schedule and is very satisfied.

Orville's mom has a chronic problem with her knee. Dr. Côté was able to help her some but unfortunately she had to return home to Jamaica as she was just staying with us for a two month visit."

Comments:

When I saw Vivienne on her first visit, her main concern was her left shoulder pain. She had consulted her doctor but the only answer for her after x-ray findings and exams was medication which helped only temporarily.

My chiropractic exam showed some limitations in shoulder movements and also a very uneven pelvis low on the left. A Surface EMG showed a significant increase in activity on the right side of the lumbar spine. All this along with her postural exam seem to explain why her secondary concerns of left hip and knee pain were occurring. With the Activator Methods assessment a misalignment in her left acromio-clavicular (AC) joint was easily found and adjusted. By the next visit, she experienced relief from the shoulder pain that had been persisting for six months.

After a few more visits she started to feel her hip and knee improve also. Even secondary problems proved to go away in time and with appropriate posture exercises and maintaining a good spine through chiropractic she stays pain free and healthy.

Care Plan:

Viviene came for three visits initially and now is on a two-month check-up schedule. The problem with her shoulder was found after a few visits but her hip and knee concerns took a few more weeks to improve.

Thought to Ponder:

What can you do for a pessimist who complains about the noise when opportunity comes knocking?

"Delays have dangerous ends."

William Shakespeare

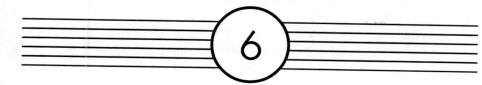

Connecting with the Office

How to Become Comfortable
with Your Health Care Partnership

Well, you have finally made the decision. You have picked up the phone, heard a pleasant, helpful voice at the other end and booked your first chiropractic appointment. Going from no action to some action always seems the most difficult. But there – it's done!

Our First Date

What can you expect when you show up for the first visit? I can only talk about my own office but I would assume your experience would be similar in other chiropractors' offices. Your initial task is to fill out a few forms to provide personal data and record your health concerns. Complete these forms with as much detail as possible even though some questions might not seem related to your problem.

In our office, if you have time to wait you can find useful chiropractic information to watch on our TV screen or pertinent tidbits in our reading material. Preliminary questions can also be answered by anyone at the front desk. For example, have you heard of Piriformis Syndrome? The TV screen will explain that it is pain in your lower buttocks from a muscle becoming too tight or in spasm. The constant or intermittent pain (not sciatica) is often caused by long distance driving.

Next, you'll have the opportunity to meet your chiropractor. Here are a few questions to keep in mind as you make a first encounter. This part of the consultation allows you to get to know and begin to trust this new person.

1. Do you like this professional? Is he/she warm and friendly?
2. Are you able to share your problems freely? Does the chiropractor listen well and comprehend what you are describing?
3. Is the doctor helpful and patient with you? How does he/she respond when you ask for an explanation?
4. Is the chiropractor a good communicator? Can you make sense of what has been explained? Does this doctor use too many big words related to chiropractic that have no meaning for you?
5. Is the person that referred you to this chiropractor happy and positive about their own experience?
6. Does the office look clean and well organized?
7. Are the staff members helpful?

The consultation provides the chiropractor an opportunity to gather as much information as possible about your concerns. Again, be as precise and concise as you can. Questions will be asked such as the location of the pain, how it feels, when it started, what caused it. Any background information is helpful for a good diagnosis; a connection will likely become clearer as you go.

An examination will follow to verify if your problem can be helped or if you should seek other health care avenues. Postural evaluations, muscle testing, motion or static palpation (feel by touch) of the spine, surface electromyography, thermography, and x-rays can be used in this step. All these tests are not necessarily done in every case. It depends on the condition being treated and its severity. The chiropractor will choose the most appropriate ones.

Often the test results will need to be analyzed to determine the best possible recommendations. You may be scheduled for a second visit to discuss the findings. You then can decide if you wish to pursue chiropractic for your problem and your care could begin that day. Occasionally when x-rays are not necessary and further analysis is not required, you may get started right away.

Your First Adjustment

The technique I generally use is the Activator Methods. During an adjustment you will be slowly lowered on a motorized table from a vertical to a horizontal position, face down. Your leg lengths will be checked repeatedly to find unevenness signifying muscle compensations in certain areas. This helps determine which areas need attention and correction. The Activator instrument delivers a force that can be aimed in different directions from various points on the bone. The adjustments are safe, specific and comfortable. Findings are recorded along with how you feel and particulars of the last few days. In chiropractic school a student learns to take "SOAP" notes which is an acronym for Subjective (how the patient is feeling), Objective (what the chiropractor observes), Assessment (evaluation) and Plan (recommendation).

Remarkably without you moving your body, the actual length of your legs will even up as appropriate adjustments are made. The objective is to get them exactly even and on each appointment thereafter find a reduced difference between the lengths. This is an indication of fewer muscle compensations and therefore less misalignments or subluxations. Bear in mind this leg length variation is due to uneven muscular tension, not a bony difference that would be impossible to change. This inequality may be as much an inch (2.5 cm) initially but then only 1/4 (.63 cm) or 1/8 (.32 cm) of an inch on following visits. To get the fastest and most effective results you should be checked every other day until your leg lengths remain very close to even at which point you should start to feel much better. The norm is a recommendation for continuing adjustments three times a week over a four week period. A good response for symptom relief can be expected between two to eight weeks.

When I examine for misalignments, I am looking for a vertebra in your spinal column that for some reason (e.g. strain, stress, wear and tear) has shifted into a wrong position. It is causing neural and joint disturbances in the area. The thrust delivered from the instrument forces this vertebra to move. The muscles reset around the vertebrae and tension in the muscles changes which evens out your leg lengths. You may have one or more subluxations, associated with pain or not, that need to be reduced. If these are not corrected the nerve messages that travel between the brain and the corresponding tissues will be disturbed.

Subluxations may be traced back to trauma having occurred years before, sometimes as early as during the birth process. This can be a stressful event for a newborn with its fragile, tiny neck especially if forceps or suction have to be used in delivery. Even such activities as learning to walk can result in repeated little upsets. Watch a baby take his or her first steps. During the ensuing weeks, how many times will this child fall? My guess would be one to two hundred times. Could this be the cause of the first misalignment? Very likely. Learning to skate or snowboard is a similar grown-up version of this type of trauma. Falling on your behind doesn't feel very good; it is never quite symmetrical. Could this also result in misalignments in your structure? Most definitely.

Paying Attention

Throughout this book you are reading testimonials from many of my patients who have found relief from a particular ailment through chiropractic care. Is your story or the story of one of your family members similar? Check out the health conditions listed in Appendix I that have been helped through chiropractic care. You might be surprised at the variety. It is particularly important to get a chiropractic assessment immediately after a physical or mental trauma such as car accidents, death of a loved one, moving, falling, shovelling to make sure no misalignments occurred and to prevent future problems from them.

Does your work insurance plan cover chiropractic expenses? Some employees don't know if it is in their benefits' package. Check out the details of your plan or ask a supervisor for information. If you are not covered, many chiropractic offices will organize an easy payment plan for you. If it is a job related injury, a worker's compensation plan (WSIB in Canada) will cover your costs. Many studies have shown that employees return to work sooner when they go to chiropractors than when using other avenues. If a chiropractor is the first health care person you see after your incident, you will not need a referral from a physician as chiropractors are primary contact health professionals. Car insurance companies also cover chiropractic for injuries from car accidents. Fill out the appropriate form to qualify and seek help within a certain time period.

Finally there is a percentage of patients who have no coverage and pay out of pocket because they realize the value of chiropractic care for them and their families. They see that staying healthy this way is cheaper in the long run than managing disease and sickness with drugs and surgery later on, not to mention the expense of time lost at work for health problems.

Check Out Your Loved Ones at Home

1. At home you can do your own version of our leg length analysis on someone else. Have your family member wear a pair of hard soled shoes and lie across a bed, face down, with arms relaxed at each side. Keep the head straight down. Apply equal pressure with both thumbs to the arches

of each shoe. Are both legs equal in length when the bottoms of the shoes are parallel or is one leg shorter than the other? A perceivable difference is significant. It is a common sign of muscle compensations from spinal problems. This is just a screening test so a check-up is probably warranted. Your chiropractor is trained to accurately pick up these differences and more.

2. To determine abnormalities in posture use a yardstick. View front and side angles as the person stands against a wall. Are the ears, shoulders, and hips uneven? Does the head lean forward? If a female (or a Scotsman who wears a kilt!), measure the distance of the hem of the skirt from the floor. Do the measurements vary from side to side? Let your chiropractor check for more accuracy if you notice something.

3. Uneven weight distribution is another good home test. Obtain two bath-room scales. Make sure both weight-bearing surfaces are level. With shoes off, tilt the head up and down, left and right, settling to a neutral position. Record the scale readings for each side. If there is an obvious difference between the two scales a professional evaluation should be pursued.

4. Check the bottom of a person's shoes. Do you see uneven wear on the soles? Similar to detecting unevenness on your car tires, irregular shoe wear could indicate a misaligned structure, an uneven gait or stance.

5. Does this person experience stiffness in the morning? The body heals itself during the night. When there is not much to heal you should be fine upon rising. When something is amiss in one's alignment causing friction or wear and tear, then more tissues need to be repaired. Stiffness may be felt in the morning after six or seven hours of healing time when scar tissue can develop. My regular patients often report they are not sore but when checked it is very common to find some structural problem occurring.

You Are Not Alone

If all this is new to you as you consider your first chiropractic visit and you feel just a little uncertain, please be assured that this is how most new patients feel. I am totally confident that if you give yourself a chance you will realize how much benefit you can gain by including chiropractic care in your life. A most frequent comment heard in our office from patients who waited a long time to connect with a chiropractor is, "I wish I had done this years ago!"

Small Troubles — Big Solutions

Name: .... Wendy Carter
From: .... Brampton, Ontario
Treated for: .... Hip Pain; Knee
                     Pain; Thumb Pain;
                     Bunion;
                     Indigestion

"Chiropractic care with Dr. Côté has taught me that I can expect a lot more from my body than I used to believe. I first visited Dr. Côté's office over 12 years ago upon the recommendation of a friend when I had fallen on my left knee on my icy driveway. My family doctor had informed me that my knee was fine – no broken bones – but it still was bothering me and so was my hip. Apparently the misalignment of my knee was throwing my hip out as well along with added repeated irritation produced from driving a gearshift car. This took a while to figure out. Today I do not have any more hip problems but I still suffer with discomfort in my knee which does improve with each adjustment and the added support of wearing a 1½ inch knee brace as recommended by Dr. Côté. Last spring during my annual check-up, my family doctor did take an x-ray of my knee and learned that my cartilage had been torn probably at the time of my fall.

With good nutritional supplements and regular chiropractic treatments I very seldom have a headache which I had experienced for many years. I enjoy gardening and when my thumb begins to throb because of the overuse of gardening shears, I know I need an adjustment to my hand. I have always believed that since my mother and my aunt had bunions on their feet that I would too. I did develop one on my right foot. After mentioning that problem to Dr. Côté a few months ago, I now remember to take my shoe off at the end of my session with her for these treatments are helping. My last question was about indigestion which I have suffered with lately. She gave me an adjustment on my stomach and recommended deep breathing from the diaphragm for ten minutes each evening. This will force my stomach further down and keep acidity from coming up the esophagus. That makes sense.

I no longer take my body for granted. If I encounter a problem there must be a solution to discover. I cannot accept the answer, 'It's only birthdays!' as suggested by my doctor at one point. Why live with discomfort when you don't have to?"

Comments:
Wendy came to my office because she was experiencing lower back pain. It wasn't severe but it was starting to interfere with her daily tasks and she wasn't too happy about that. As an afterthought, she mentioned she had fallen in her driveway and injured her left knee in doing so. She said that it had never been the same since.

Her exam, x-rays and Surface EMG test seemed to indicate that her lower back pain was secondary to the left knee injury as she seemed to be standing deviated to the right as though trying to take her weight off the left side. Going with that premise after realigning her lower back, I made sure her left knee was also realigned. She progressed quickly and was able to resume her regular activities with ease and comfort.

Wendy's satisfaction with chiropractic care through the years comes more from the fact that she can remain active and productive than being completely pain free. She does get into trouble occasionally from doing too much but getting adjusted is an answer for that.

Care Plan:
Wendy came three times a week initially and now visits once every six weeks.

Sports Minded

Name: .... Adrienne Gittens
From: .... Mississauga, Ontario
Treated for: .... Shoulder Pain; Knee Injury

"My husband, Anthony, introduced me to the science of chiropractic. He has had neck and back problems all his life due to a muscle that was damaged by forceps during his birth. We were managing a bakery. Anthony was in need of an adjustment so he located the chiropractors that owned the practice that Dr. Côté purchased.

Due to the constant rolling of dough for our bakery goods, I began having problems with my shoulder. After my husband's encouragement when I couldn't move my shoulder, I became a patient around 1984 in the Erindale Chiropractic Clinic. I didn't know much about chiropractic back then but I was willing to learn and even joined the staff in 1991 as a Chiropractic Assistant after Dr. Côté became the new owner. It was normal for chiropractors at this time to have their patients initially visit their offices three times a week for six weeks, then two times a week for six weeks and then once a week for six weeks. Dr. Côté acquainted me with the Activator method which results, it seems, in a shorter time frame for improvement.

Today Dr. Côté checks me every ten days or so as I like to play tennis three times a week and my body is getting older. A few years ago I hurt my knee while playing tennis and chiropractic care has made a tremendous difference in my ability to continue playing my favourite sport two or three times a week without after affects and without medication. In the meantime my knowledge of chiropractic has grown through lots of reading and listening to tapes available in our office.

I loved my position as Dr. Côté's Office Manager for many years. We saw a lot of success with babies that have suffered with colic. After a couple of adjustments the babies are more relaxed and the colic disappears. It was also exciting to see patients relieved from the throbbing pain of sciatica. Even though patients come and go – some return as regulars and some don't – I have found that those that continue to return, as I did, benefit from a higher level of health."

Comments:

Adrienne is a perfect example of someone who leads a chiropractic health style kind of life. Without getting into the age thing, let's just say she has four grandchildren, works full time, plays tennis, and doesn't need medication for anything.

If there is a knee and hip complaint occasionally she gets adjusted and recovers. Whenever she is stressed physically, chemically or mentally her first action is to get an adjustment before anything starts to hurt. This minimizes the need for acute care which is more trying for the patient and the chiropractor because the patient is upset.

I have noticed through the years that her spinal alignment has been improving instead of worsening with age. It is a very noticeable and measurable improvement that could only happen with chiropractic care.

Care Plan:
Adrienne came initially three times a week for six weeks, then two times a week for six weeks and then once a week for six weeks. Her current maintenance plan is every ten days or so.

Thought to Ponder:

Do ex-politicians become devoted?

"The greatest mistake physicians make is that they attempt to cure the body without attempting to cure the mind; yet the mind and body are one and should not be treated separately."

Plato

7

Connecting with Others
How a Government Report Views Chiropractic

Awell-formed team with each player contributing in the best way possible leads to the best experience. The team performs as one. Throughout the reading of this book you have caught a bit of my heart, passion and objectives. I could not run my practice smoothly without relying on excellent staff that manages such daily tasks as accounting, reception, purchasing. I am very thankful for the assistants that surround me as their enthusiasm, cheerfulness and loyalty is what is needed to better care for my patients.

Team Captain

Another big component in making this team work is you. When you visit my office you are at least showing me that you are willing to try. Chiropractic is not new but it might be very new to you. Some patients who arrive in my office lack any hope that I can make a difference for them. Do you remember my saying earlier on that my father loved to make people laugh? Do you remember his "keep smiling" signs around his office? In similar fashion and following through on Plato's advice (on opposite page), having a positive attitude will make a difference in how you respond.

Keep things light; don't take yourself too seriously. One patient has been struggling with a torn cartilage in her left knee. She really doesn't want surgery and so I have been adjusting her knee. One day I suggested she wear a brace just below the knee cap for support. It was proving quite successful until one day while out gardening for an hour she realized she had put the brace on the wrong leg. We all got a good laugh over that one. At least she was brave enough to share her blunder with others.

It has probably taken a while for you to get into this uncomfortable condition. Believe that it will take some time for your body to be restored to where you want it to be. Follow through on any instructions given. Take home the brochures available to become more informed. Take charge of your life to improve your situation rather than lethargically accept the way it is. You are part of the solution.

More Team Members

When you become a satisfied patient, will you talk about your recovery to your family and friends? Share your personal experience with them. Give them a copy of this book for better understanding of chiropractic. They will be ever so grateful that you took this initiative and you will feel good about yourself for helping them out. Do you remember B.J. Palmer's desire to have the word "chiropractic" become a household word? Maybe together we can accomplish that goal in our lifetime.

Also, please do not be afraid to mention your new care plan to your family doctor. Quite often these days, your physician will encourage you to continue with your plan of recovery because it is successful. Share your story with your M.D. Remember medical doctors might not know very much about what chiropractors do. And they definitely don't have extra time to "bone" (another pun intended!) up on it with their very busy schedules. By recommending chiropractic more, doctors could lighten the load on the health care systems and have extra time to deal with true medical emergencies. But first they have to know the positive effects chiropractic care has on their patients. I truly think that patients sharing their success stories with their doctors more frequently could accomplish that.

Good Team Effort

The following chart summarizes well how your experience in a chiropractor's office can be greatly enhanced. It takes "two to tango!"

The Chiropractor's Job

1. See you as a person, not a condition.
2. Respect your privacy and your time.
3. Provide a comfortable office setting.
4. Explain procedures and findings.
5. Monitor and report your progress.
6. Show you ways to get and stay well.
7. Offer state-of-the-art chiropractic.
8. Refer to other specialists as needed.
9. Charge a fair fee for services.
10. Honor your individual health goals.

The Patient's Job

1. Want better health.
2. Get involved.
3. Keep appointments.
4. Follow advice.
5. Ask questions.
6. Seek answers.
7. Expect results.
8. Stay optimistic.
9. Pay your bills.
10. Tell others.

The Manga Report

There have been several noteworthy chiropractic studies and reports compiled throughout the years by teams of researchers. One such important study from 1993 was ordered and funded by the Ontario Ministry of Health called "The Effectiveness and Cost-Effectiveness of Chiropractic Management of Low-Back Pain."

This study was headed up by Pran Manga, Ph. D. As a university professor from Ottawa, ON, his specialty is health administration and especially health economics. On more than 40 occasions he has served as a consultant to Canadian governments. To be perfectly clear, he is not a chiropractor; he is an objective analyst who took a hard look at all the facts about how the government could save billions of dollars in the area of managing lower back pain. The Ontario government, not chiropractors, sponsored this study because of the rising costs of managing lower back pain in the health care system. In addition, there is a tremendous cost to the economy with sick time used by people staying home from work because of lower back pain.

It is important to understand that in Ontario where I reside there is a prior commitment to maintaining a health care system which is publicly funded with tax dollars. OHIP is an acronym for Ontario Health Insurance Plan – the government funded health care system in Ontario.

Carefully look at the following highlights from the Manga Report Executive Summary listed below. Ask yourself how anyone could reject such compelling conclusions founded on objective facts. Even though these conclusions were made back in 1993, there is nothing to suggest the situation is any different today or will be 50 years from now.

Highlighted Findings:

(Please note that LBP = lower back pain)[15]

1. On the evidence, particularly the most scientifically valid clinical studies, spinal manipulation applied by chiropractors is shown to be more effective than alternative treatments for LBP. Many medical therapies are of questionable validity or are clearly inadequate.

2. There is no clinical or case-control study that demonstrates or even implies that chiropractic spinal manipulation is unsafe in the treatment of low-back pain. Some medical treatments are equally safe, but others are unsafe and generate iatrogenic complications for LBP patients. Our reading of the literature suggests that chiropractic manipulation is safer than medical management of low-back pain.

3. ...several existing medical therapies of LBP are generally contraindicated on the basis of the existing clinical trials. There is also some evidence in the literature to suggest that spinal manipulations are less safe and less effective when performed by non-chiropractic professionals.

4. There is an overwhelming body of evidence indicating that chiropractic management of low-back pain is more cost-effective than medical management.

5. There would be highly significant cost savings if more management of LBP was transferred from physicians to chiropractors. Evidence from Canada and other countries suggests potential savings of many hundreds of millions annually...Workers' Compensation studies report that injured workers with the same specific diagnosis of LBP returned to work much sooner when treated by chiropractors than by physicians.

6. There is good empirical evidence that patients are very satisfied with chiropractic management of LBP and considerably less satisfied with physician management.

7. ...the use of chiropractic has grown steadily over the years. Chiropractors are now accepted as a legitimate healing profession by the public and an increasing number of physicians.

8. a) the effectiveness and cost-effectiveness of chiropractic management of low-back pain,

   b) the untested, questionable or harmful nature of many current medical therapies,

   c) the economic efficiency of chiropractic care for low-back pain compared with medical care,

   d) the safety of chiropractic care,

   e) the higher satisfaction levels expressed by patients of chiropractors,

   together offers an overwhelming case in favor of much greater use of chiropractic services in the management of low-back pain.

9. The government will have to instigate and monitor the reform called for by our overall conclusions, and take appropriate steps to see that the savings are captured. The greater use of chiropractic services in the health care delivery system will not occur by itself, ...

Recommendations to the Government:

1. There should be a shift in policy now to encourage and prefer chiropractic services for most patients with LBP.

2. Chiropractic services should be fully insured under the Ontario Health Insurance Plan.

3. Chiropractic services should be fully integrated into the health care system.

4. Chiropractors should be employed by tertiary hospitals in Ontario.

5. Hospital privileges should be extended to all chiropractors for the purposes of treatment of their own patients who have been hospitalized for other reasons, and for access to diagnostic facilities relevant to their scope of practice and patients' needs.

6.   Chiropractors should have access to all pertinent patient records and tests from hospitals, physicians, and other health care professionals upon the consent of their patients.

7.   Since low-back pain is of such significant concern to worker's compensation, chiropractors should be engaged at a senior level by Workers' Compensation Board to assess policy, procedures and treatment of workers with back injuries... A very good case can be made for making chiropractors the gatekeepers for management of low-back pain in the workers' compensation system in Ontario.

8.   The government should make the requisite research funds and resources available for further clinical evaluation of chiropractic management of LBP and for further socioeconomic and policy research concerning the management of LBP generally.

9.   Chiropractic education in Ontario should be in the multidisciplinary atmosphere of a university with appropriate public funding.

10. The government should take all reasonable steps to actively encourage cooperation between providers, particularly the chiropractic, medical and physiotherapy professions.

Serious Savings

This report, a collection of different studies from all over the world on lower back care, was generated from Dr. Manga and his team of experts. It clearly encourages that chiropractic should be included in the complete health care lineup. This economist is adamant about the billions of dollars that could be saved every year if these changes were implemented.

Some significant passages from this report are: "The mean disability compensation paid to workers was $264 for those treated by chiropractic compared to $618 and $1565 for those treated by physicians and osteopaths respectively."

"The early return to work is an important factor in cost saving and hence the average compensation days with chiropractic management are one quarter (6.26) the days of claims with medical management (25.56)."

"Patients treated by chiropractors had significantly lower rate of compensable injury (23.2 versus 57.7 percent) when compared to physicians and osteopaths."

It was calculated that by using these strategies the savings would climb into the millions or even billions of dollars just for the care of lower back pain alone. Imagine if this thinking was extended into all the conditions chiropractic care can help. It seems to me that the savings to the health care system would be very significant, even if chiropractic care was fully funded by the government. In addition, we would have a healthier, stronger society as a result. I want to be on that kind of winning team. How about you?

Connection Story

Jaw Dropping News

Name: .... Alison Hamouth
From: .... Mississauga, Ontario
Treated for: .... Temporo Mandibular Joint (TMJ);
.... Fainting Spells; Convulsions

"My name is Lauren James. I worked at Erindale Chiropractic Clinic with Drs. Côté and Andersen for many years. I have seen all the wonders that chiropractic produces and I am no stranger to the healing qualities it brings. I was, however, knocked off my feet by what happened to my daughter, Alison.

Ali has been receiving chiropractic care since birth. When she was 15 she fainted in her gym class and landed face down. She received a whiplash type injury and required stitches to her chin. Once she hit the ground she convulsed. The witnesses said it was relatively mild. The doctors said the convulsion was probably from the fall. Ali continued to have convulsions at least once every two weeks, sometimes every few days, from then on. She remained conscious throughout each attack but would shake and she was unable to talk. The attacks would last about ten minutes after which she was exhausted and would need to sleep. You can imagine how this interfered with school and teenage life. She was not allowed to take stairs alone or cross streets by herself.

Every conceivable test was done and redone with no explanation. Finally during a neurological examination it was pointed out that Alison had what was an apparently unrelated issue with her jaw called TMJ (temporo mandibular joint or jaw disorder as evidenced by the lower and upper teeth not coming together properly while biting). The suggestion was made that maybe her dentist should take a look at it. We left the neurologist's office and went straight to see Dr. Côté instead. Yes, the TMJ was definitely out of alignment. It was adjusted and adjusted again two days later. After two adjustments it was in alignment. Alison has not had one attack since.

Quite possibly the original, unexplained fall on her chin may have caused the jaw misalignment. Coincidence? Hmmm…

Oh and by the way, I am still happily employed in the chiropractic field."

Comments:

Alison's story surprised me as much as it surprised her and her mom. I would not even attempt to explain the neurological pathways that can lead to convulsions such as she experienced.

When I examined Alison it was very obvious that her temporo mandibular joint was out of alignment and needed to be adjusted. I didn't usually find this with her on her regular visits.

One can suffer diverse symptoms from a misaligned jaw such as headaches, dizziness, facial pain, tooth pain and the obvious chewing malfunction. But seizures were new for me! Today Alison is adjusted monthly before she gets any more full blown episodes and it does wonders for her.

Care Plan:

Alison was adjusted a few times after her fall and now comes once a month for regular check-ups.

Drop the Drugs

Name: .... Joe Faria
From: .... Mississauga, Ontario
Treated For: .... Neck Pain; Lower Back Pain; Foot Pain; Sciatica; Swelling; Poor Circulation

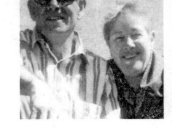

Connection Story

"One spring several years ago when I walked into Dr. Côté's chiropractic office, my symptoms were neck pain, swelling, spasms and stiffness due to osteoarthritis. I also had pain in my lower back and foot. I was suffering with these extremely severe symptoms for over a year.

I had been previously prescribed Prednisone and Voltaren drugs from specialists with nonexistent results. I discontinued the drugs due to my fear of the possible side effects.

I had no doubts chiropractic would help me. I really appreciated the gentle method of adjustment used by this doctor. She was understanding and knowledgeable. The office staff was very friendly. Within six months of treatment I became functional again. The swelling disappeared and the pain was controlled. It was like magic! Today I continue to see Dr. Côté once a month unless something comes up that requires extra treatment.

I've told my friends and family about chiropractic. Read my wife's story next. My daughter has been adjusted for her neck, upper back pain and sciatica. My grandchildren come in for maintenance care. Chiropractic has helped minimize all of their symptoms and has provided them with a general feeling of well-being.

I would recommend others try non-drug methods, modify their lifestyle and try chiropractic treatment. I've always trusted the concept of chiropractic and now that the method is gentler I feel even surer about its benefits."

Comments:
During Joe's first visit he was very calm describing his symptoms and his search for relief. He had tried everything he could think of – all the way to flying to Portugal to sit in the healing springs without success.

I remember upon my examination I was surprised to see that his left foot had become a dark purple from poor circulation. Most people think that sciatica can only be in the form of pain but often we find other neurological deficits such as numbness, weird sensations, muscle weakness and wasting, and poor circulation. I asked Joe if he had showed his doctor his purple foot and he assured me he had. The doctor didn't think anything could be done after all the crucial blocked artery tests were taken. After a few months of care, not only did Joe's neck feel better but his purple foot was now pink again.

Care Plan:
Joe had six months of treatment two to three times a week initially to overcome most of his symptoms and now visits our office once a month for maintenance.

That Feels Better

Name: .... Paulina Faria
From: .... Mississauga, Ontario
Treated for: .... Neck Pain; Back Pain; Indigestion, Gas; Bloating; Stomach Pain

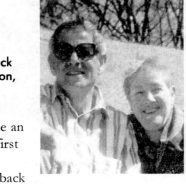

"About a year before my husband made an appointment with Dr. Côté, I was the first to consult her regarding two distinct problems. I had been having neck and back pain constantly for years. I was also experiencing indigestion, gas, bloating and stomach pain with every meal.

Various antacids and fibre supplements provided temporary relief for the digestive problems. Yoga provided good results for the neck and back problem when I was consistent.

Five years previously I had tried chiropractic and had not found it helpful. I had heard good things from my friends that had received help with the use of the Activator method. They convinced me to try chiropractic again. I was thrilled about the gentle method, friendly staff and attentive, concerned doctor. I now experience no pain in the neck or back and the digestion has improved dramatically.

I would suggest for others who are sick, suffering, or in pain to be open-minded. Try natural methods such as chiropractic before getting involved with drugs. Read up on your condition. Get fit. Think positive. I've told many friends and family about chiropractic. I recommend it!"

Comments:

Paulina came to my office at first for intense pain in her arms, some upper back pain, lower back pain and occasional shooting pains down her legs.

Chiropractic care helped her tremendously and within a month of adjusting her lower back disc and her cervical spine she was ready to exercise her degenerated lumbar disc. There is a specific lumbar disc exercise that we use to improve this situation. I also suggested cervical spine posture exercise to normalize the position of her neck.

Very often I will send patients home with exercises so they can participate in improving certain things such as posture and flexibility.

Connection Story

Sometimes relearning how to walk properly is necessary after chronic pelvic problems. Other times proper breathing techniques need to be taught to avoid rib injuries or poor digestion. Better ways to sit or lie need to be discussed occasionally or anything that might put undue strain on the spine.

This is an important part of chiropractic care as an educated patient is a healthier patient and one that is less likely to injure themselves with regular daily activities.

Care Plan:

Paulina had several adjustments three times a week for one month and then we gradually decreased the frequency of visits to once a month. She remains on this plan.

Thought to Ponder:

**If you have x-ray vision and could
see through everything,
would you see anything at all?**

**"Be brave as your fathers before you.
Have faith and go forward."**

Thomas Edison

8

Connecting with the Future

How to Change Your World So Your Family and Friends Can Enjoy Better Lives

The famous quote, "I have a dream ..." from Martin Luther's passionate speech on August 28, 1963 is recognized by most people. It is amazing how the power of his vision altered our world. Parts of his dream are now a reality and the world is a better place because of it.

I also have a dream – a vision for a better health care system; one that is gentle, safe and natural; one that could be immeasurably less costly, more effective and more accessible. It is a health care system that includes chiropractic care in all aspects of neuro-musculoskeletal health from the moment of birth to the day we die. I envision a health care system that is aimed at improving people's health by preventing problems before they occur. I dream of people having choices on how they take care of their own health and that of their families.

An Integrated Health Care System

What would this perfect health care system look like? For me, it would consist of the development and reevaluation of two areas – record-keeping and multidisciplinary services included in hospital emergency wards, walk-in clinics and private health care offices.

First of all, I have realized over my years as a chiropractor, we health care professionals do not communicate or consult very often with each other. We do not share scientific data from old and new research. We don't even report to each other on the progress of our mutual patients. Every health care discipline seems to work on its own, whether it is family medicine, chiropractic, massage therapy, naturopathy etc. Secondly, our hospital emergency rooms need dire changes because of major problems such as wait times, appropriateness of care and follow-up.

Electronic Health Records

Here's an idea to facilitate exchange of information among health care workers. Each patient would have an electronic health record bank saved on whatever medium is used at the time and kept in a safe, confidential place. This data would be accessible by scanning the person's digital prints or retina. (This is for all the Trekkies out there!) Personal information gathered in this bank would include details of birth, childhood diseases, recurrent health problems while growing up, medications prescribed or any other interventions undertaken such as surgeries. Alternative health care procedures and diagnoses such professionals as naturopaths, chiropractors, physiotherapists, or podiatrists would also be recorded here.

Positive Benefits

Imagine how much safer such a system would be for patients as records of all medication taken are kept in one place for all doctors to consider. Since side effects would be documented it would be obvious what medication a person should avoid in the future. This would also help to prevent mixing medications that should not be combined.

Imagine the possible millions of dollars saved when this type of documentation is readily available. There would be fewer repeated tests or procedures as tests already done could be made readily available to any health care professional that the patient would consult.

Imagine the possibilities in research if everybody's information could be used anonymously. Response to all types of care would become available and could help evaluate the effectiveness and at the same time discern possible dangers of different health care approaches.

Imagine the efficiency of having your entire detailed health history on an electronic file. You wouldn't have to repeat or try to recall your story every time you saw someone for a health concern. I can also see us using these records for preliminary consultations. You could send them to your chosen health practitioners and see if, based on your symptoms and your electronic records, they would have strategies to help you. You could then arrange an actual consultation with the approach that resonates the most with you.

For example, if you had a sore leg and decided that you wanted your medical doctor, your chiropractor and a physiotherapist to address your problem, you could send your health records to each of them along with a description of your present symptoms. They would automatically have access to all the tests, x-rays and procedures done for you to this point. They would also have a complete history of how and when this problem started along with a detailed history of all your injuries throughout your life. These professionals would respond with their possible diagnoses and recommendations for your problem. Then you could make an educated decision on how you would want your health dollars spent.

Simplified Choices

For patients everywhere this could simplify choosing where to go for help especially in remote areas as you would be more sure that you are going to the right place for your particular problem. It would also cut down on many unnecessary consultations.

Here is an illustration of how important electronic records can be. One day a young boy, Kyle, whom I had been seeing for years, came in with fairly severe left calf pain. I checked him over, found a few things out of alignment, corrected them and had him return two days later. During Kyle's second visit, it was obvious he was still very sore. He could hardly put weight on his left leg and when I rechecked him I found nothing out of alignment. His leg was now swollen, red and hot. I immediately sent Kyle to his medical doctor. A blood clot was found in his leg causing the pain. It was evident that when I checked him the second time there was something else wrong; a quick referral was the appropriate action. An electronic personal health record bank in this instance would have been so handy for me and his doctor. Exchange of information would have been faster, easier and more effective.

There is much to be excited about as this technology is right at our fingertips. Improved safety for patients, better efficiency for health care workers and better opportunities for research for our scientists would be the outcome of keeping records this way.

A Difficult Night

I recently spent a very difficult night in a hospital emergency room with my 15 year old son, Max, and let me tell you that I found it to be a very disturbing experience. I feel very blessed that my family and I are generally very healthy in that if we are ill we have alternative options.

We were very tired as it was 3 a.m. The waiting room was overflowing with people seeking help. Some were moaning in extreme pain, others vomiting into plastic buckets while others were coughing incessantly or crying for attention. It was an awful situation to say the least. As we waited our turn to see the doctor (only one on staff), we tried to catch some shut-eye. Sleep was next to impossible sitting on uncomfortable vinyl chairs under harsh lights and surrounded with constant loud noises. The hospital staff were tired, insensitive and overworked trying to serve the needs of an overcrowded waiting room.

A healthy person having to tolerate all this for any length of time would become sick themselves. I know I almost was and unlike some who had been there even longer, our wait was a mere five hours before we saw the doctor. Bear in mind that we were in the rapid assessment zone as my son with a swollen tonsil couldn't swallow, drink, eat or even breathe through his mouth at that point. What about others in not so critical waiting zones? I hear my patients tell similar stories much too often.

Finally the person ahead of us was seen. She lay in the next bed to us behind a thin curtain so unfortunately I could hear what brought her in for this emergency visit. Her neck was sore and she was experiencing muscle spasms in her upper back which got worse when she took a deep breath. This is a common complaint heard in our offices and one that can often respond well in most cases with chiropractic care. This lady could have been cared for by a chiropractor immediately or sent to her own chiropractor the next day. Instead she took 30 minutes of the doctor's valuable time, had to undergo x-rays and wait for the results in that waiting room that I'm sure most of us would rather avoid. She probably was given a prescription for pain killers and muscle relaxants and sent home being no further ahead than the day before. Meanwhile people were still throwing up in the waiting room.

Suggested Changes

Here is how I envision a friendlier, warmer atmosphere in our emergency rooms. The waiting rooms would be set up as little oases of peace and serenity. The harsh lights would be replaced by more subdued lighting. There would be calming sounds like rain falling, birds chirping or classical music playing. The chairs would be comfortable enough to rest or even sleep on if need be. Patients would be kept informed on the status of their wait so they could plan a bathroom break, get a drink or inform their workplace or family members about their situation.

A medical doctor would continue to look after emergencies, of course; but a chiropractor and a naturopath would assist as well. Patients could then be triaged more appropriately and efficiently to save time. Our lady with the neck problem would probably be seen by the chiropractor, had x-rays taken and sent with a referral to see her own chiropractor the next day if it was warranted. There would be collaboration between the three doctors on the floor so that the best care would be given to each patient.

This multidisciplinary approach could also be reproduced in walk-in or private health care clinics. My office complex includes a naturopath, a chiropodist, massage therapists in addition to chiropractic services. This configuration has proven very beneficial many times for me, my associates and our patients.

Womb to Tomb

Before reaching an emergency status it is possible that most health problems could be avoided or even eliminated if chiropractic were integrated into every facet of life. From our first breath to our last moment, I see chiropractic care being the initial line of action when a malfunction occurs.

The birth of a baby is a natural process; it is not a health problem, nor usually an emergency. I believe we should interfere with it as little as possible. I envision midwives working closely with chiropractors, naturopaths, dieticians and personal trainers during pregnancy and after delivery. Midwives know when medical attention is required so that expensive medical care and procedures would only be used when absolutely necessary. Deliveries would occur at home wherever advisable and practical.

I was very happy with my "at home" experience when our son, Max, was born (Julie was delivered in the hospital due to breech complications). My midwife was wonderful. I truly believe a home birth is the way to go for a normal pregnancy. The hospital bed that is freed up could be used for emergencies.

After Max was born, the midwives had left and everybody was finally asleep, I remember sneaking downstairs to the kitchen to make myself a peanut butter sandwich. The luxury of that moment is very difficult to explain but one that I will always remember. Overall it was a very positive experience. How many women can say the same these days about their deliveries?

I see a chiropractor assisting midwives during the birth process in a home environment or birthing centers if accessible. He would check the mother before and after birth for spinal misalignments. The newborn would also be checked soon after the birth to ensure that this baby would have the best structural ad neurological health possible.

Midwives give the baby and the family unit personalized attention from conception to a few months after the happy arrival. Every baby needs to get off to a good start with the least amount of trauma possible and with the most natural nutrition – breast-feeding. This is what midwives focus on and enable.

Under midwives' care, everyone in the family is considered and supported throughout the whole pregnancy process. After delivery the midwives visit their clients' homes to help with such problems as postpartum depression, colicky babies, nursing difficulties, sleeping problems, baby's skin problems and even those occasional troubles with sibling rivalries. Most of these concerns can be addressed by midwives successfully which can often avoid extra costly medical care. Consider the cost savings if even half the births occurred this way.

In the health care system I long for, most people would begin life this way. They would have access to gentle chiropractic care during and right after the birth process. This would avoid the first possible structural problem that can occur and therefore allow the best possible start for their nervous system.

Childhood

Early on, the baby would be checked when spinal curvatures are formed. This happens when baby starts to hold its head up. When the baby begins to crawl, to sit and then walk, chiropractic check-ups allow for normal spinal curve development. The young child doesn't need to have pain to make sure all is developing as it should.

A growing child would be checked regularly whenever a stressor, whether mechanical, mental or chemical, occurred. After traumas, falls, hits from sports, bad posture and emotional stresses children would be checked to make sure that their structure and nervous system are not compromised. Nutritional evaluation would help improve the child's diet with counseling given on what should be consumed to remain healthy. Such advice would include information on extra supplements or avoidance of certain foods. In this way naturopaths and dieticians would be invaluable to a child's health.

Dental care would continue in much the same way. This profession has done a great job educating the public on the hygiene of teeth so they can keep them for life. Isn't it just as important to keep your spine and nervous system healthy for life?

Adulthood

Following good early childhood attention, many structural problems and ensuing health problems could be prevented. Then in adulthood, with a well functioning nervous system, people would only need occasional chiropractic check-ups depending on their type of job, stress levels and environment. They wouldn't need to wait for malfunction or pain to dictate care. All chiropractors have measurement methods to find subluxations even before symptoms occur. It is obviously beneficial to handle these subluxations as early as possible.

Furthermore, studies have shown that adjustments can boost white blood cell formation and strengthen the immune system. Patients with a possible immune system weakness would receive chiropractic. This could help them better fight infectious diseases whether viral, bacterial or fungal. For this same reason those with autoimmune diseases such as diabetes, multiple sclerosis, rheumatoid arthritis, lupus would be looked after by their chiropractors in addition to their doctors.

Patients in chiropractic offices would be shown the value of good posture and the ways to strive for it in all their activities. They would be educated on the proper ways of sitting, standing and sleeping. I find it surprising how many people are not aware of what is good posture. For example, I have seen patients with chronic hip problems who have confessed that their favorite sitting position is with one leg tucked under them. It will not surprise you that the bad hip is usually the one that is tucked under. Others with similar hip problems are continually crossing their legs while sitting. If this habit is more comfortable with the same leg always crossed over the other, then this could be a sign that your pelvis is uneven and distorted. There are also many stomach sleepers out there not realizing that their chronic headaches or migraines may very well result from the fact that their heads are twisted to one side for hours during the night. How can a cervical spine stay in good alignment in such a position?

A little effort to make changes in your daily habits could help tremendously in your overall health and even prevent some of those unwanted aches and pains.

Living Longer

When these changes become reality, health challenges would be managed earlier and at a fraction of the present cost. As each and every adult would have regular chiropractic check-ups they would avoid many problems that cause pain. This could drastically decrease the need for prescribed pain medication and work sick days.

It is easy to imagine a decrease in our death rate. When fewer people need to go to the hospital for treatment or take potent medication with its inherent side effects, there is less chance to suffer bad complications. As well, mistakes can happen all too often in the higher risk medical care system. Almost everybody knows of a death that occurred because of mistakes made in the hospital or following a drug reaction.

Aging would happen gradually without the need for various medications. A well aligned spine and a good working nervous system should be sufficient to keep most people healthy and active. I see examples of that every day in my office with my regular patients.

One elderly lady retorted that half the stuff in her shopping cart these days is labeled "for fast relief." We all want fast relief and I know that chiropractic more often than not can provide that longed for result sooner than other medical avenues. If everyone used chiropractic care the way I envision it, chronic pain would be rare.

Reduced Wait Times

As fewer people require services from medical doctors or hospitals, wait times for emergencies or surgeries would decrease. These providers, in turn, would have more time and energy to offer to their patients.

In instances where physicians or specialists could not come up with a solution to a patient's health problem, chiropractors would be consulted to see if this particular health problem fell into the structural and nervous system category. Neither doctors nor chiropractors know everything; but as a team we could be much more effective.

Cost Control

Medical costs are sky rocketing. You can only begin to imagine the huge expense of hospital stays, fancy tests, nurse and doctor salaries just to name a few. Even with all this money spent sometimes answers cannot be found for patients. Alternatively if patients were screened properly initially some would be directed towards chiropractic care for answers with incredible cost savings.

Here's one of many examples. A patient of mine practiced as a nurse. She hurt her neck badly trying to lift a patient. This injury resulted in a herniated disk in of her cervical spine. She started to suffer from terrible neck and right arm pain afterward. Her doctor and many specialists concurred that surgery was not an option because of the risk factor. Medication was the treatment of choice.

When I first saw this lady she had been in pain for two years and on three different potent pain killers. She was unable to work and look after her eight-year old son as she would have liked. After a few months of chiropractic care she improved by 90% and was able to get rid of all pain killers. If chiropractic had been her first option instead of the last one, how many tens of thousands of dollars could have been saved, not to mention her job and unthinkable pain and suffering.

New New New

The chiropractic scientific community is always coming up with new ways of evaluating the nervous system. New tools of measurement are being developed. For example, thermography determines small variances in skin temperature. With thermography we can measure the temperature on both sides of the spine at one level. A considerable difference between both sides could indicate a problem with the sympathetic nervous system. If you recall from chapter four one of the jobs of this portion of the nervous system is to control blood flow to the skin. A significant difference in temperature at one spinal level can give us insight on how effectively the sympathetic nervous system is functioning.

Surface electromyography is another testing procedure that can indicate if there has been nerve interference affecting the function of the muscles on either side of the spine. The level of electrical activity can be quite different on either side if there is a problem. The HRV (Heart Rate Variability) test can also give us information on the autonomic nervous system function by measuring the heart beat timing and how quickly it varies to changes in demand. Lower heart variability means a less healthy response because of less effective neurological control. These testing procedures are quick, painless and inexpensive.

In the future other tests will eventually be used to measure health levels in patients. For example, in a recent study long term chiropractic care has been shown to influence blood serum thiol levels. This substance is a marker for DNA repair enzyme activity and therefore can be used as a measure of human health status. Higher levels of serum thiol indicate higher levels of health and a less active disease process. Please see Appendix II to read more about this study.

The future is indeed bright when you look at health care with a chiropractor's perspective. With all these scientific advances becoming available to detect problems and increased integration of this natural and safe health care, you will no doubt be benefiting immeasurably.

Another Example from My Family

Because of chiropractic care and our health philosophy, my family uses the medical system as a last resort. I estimate on average we spend less than $1000 a year for the four of us. Many years we have spent nothing. Other times there have been a few emergencies that have required our use of it. One year I broke my arm and my son, Max, when younger, suffered with asthma attacks. These incidents plus Max's most recent hospitalization are exceptions to the rule; to be sure I was very grateful to have medical options during these crises.

After I broke my arm, in addition to the medical attention I consulted my naturopath for nutritional advice on supplements which really helped speed up my recovery. In about three weeks I was told to start moving my arm as the two pieces of bone had mended. I also did a course of physiotherapy and shiatsu massage. And last but not least I used chiropractic care to keep everything as well aligned as possible during the healing process.

Surprisingly, I was back to work within four months. The orthopedic surgeons and specialists who had initially seen me had predicted that an injury like mine at my age would normally take at least six months to recover.

In my son Max's case, after his first hospital stay for the asthma attacks, he was sent home with two different kinds of puffers and a life sentence of asthma with its related problems. Our first course of action was to increase his chiropractic care to daily check-ups and then schedule a visit to our naturopath. Recommendations given were changes in his diet (avoiding rice, dried fruit and citrus juices), additions of certain supplements and homeopathic remedies as well as lifestyle changes – some as simple as avoiding cold and wet feet, getting rid of his bedroom carpet and using an air filter in his room. All this took more effort and money because chiropractic care and naturopathy are not covered in our health care system. However, the outcome was well worth it as our son is no longer asthmatic and doesn't require puffers and medication to function.

A Dream Producing Better Results

I know of many families who take care of their health problems similarly. What a difference it would make if even a small percentage of families organized their health care this way. Costs would be dramatically cut not to mention there would be less demand on our doctors, specialists and emergency rooms. In addition to the benefits for the patient, the outcome of using less medication would help clean the environment from the by-products of the drugs entering our water systems. Nice bonus!

These examples of improvements to our health care system seem simple and easy enough but it does require a transformation in our thinking. Isn't that the way President Barack Obama's journey started? Sometimes good changes do begin with a dream.

A Crooked Man

Name: .... Tomasz Jaszczy
From: .... Mississauga, Ontario
Treated for: .... Scoliosis

"I started off my teen years learning that I was suffering from scoliosis. My shoulders were not exactly aligned. My family doctor at first suggested I wait it out to see how it progressed.

A family member referred me to Dr. Côté. She realigned my spine and I improved at a rather quick pace which was amazing. I was so thankful that my headaches disappeared. It took a year before the pain was fully corrected which included the pain in my rib cage. I saw Dr. Côté three times a week to begin with, then two times a week until I was down to once a month.

At age 14 my family doctor had finally referred me to an orthopaedic surgeon at Sick Children's hospital in Toronto where I was prescribed a brace to wear for two years. After I stopped wearing the brace, the muscles holding up my spine were weakened. As a result, I was prone to misalignments. My back pain became severe and I had to take pain killers. My rib cage was also misaligned which caused a difficulty in breathing with symptoms similar to a heart attack. My heart palpitations were rather scary. When I went to the emergency room, the physicians thought I was having a panic attack. No panic attack but I had aching pains in my chest as a bone was protruding. To compensate for the pain I would put a pillow under my shirt just in the right position. This was the only thing that helped.

I am now in university and continue to see Dr. Côté regularly. If I do have pain I know that it is not wise for me to wait a day or two for it to go away. I must have realignment immediately with Dr. Côté using the Activator method. The pain recedes in a matter of hours and goes away within days.

I have recommended her service to others. Some have followed that advice; others have not. Some of my friends have even accompanied me to watch the adjustment which has helped dissolve their skepticism.

Chiropractic is a great influence in my life aiding me in feeling good from day to day."

Comments:

When I first saw him, Tomasz's scoliosis gave him minor aches and pains generally. After many trips to the Sick Children's Hospital (known affectionately as Sick Kids), it was decided he would wear a body brace. These devices are usually big, rigid and restrict some breathing movements. He was required to wear it as much as he could, almost around the clock. According to my notes, he had more complaints after he started wearing his second brace. He experienced more chest pain, difficulty breathing, and neck pain among other concerns.

The worst occurrence happened when he went to Poland for the summer while this brace was being worn. He had acute chest pain for the entire two months. When he returned I remember having to adjust his rib cage for these chest pains and irregular heartbeat. That, as you can imagine, made him quite anxious and tense worsening an already difficult situation. He experienced relief every time I saw him but the symptoms kept returning.

Ten months after he started with his second brace, he could dispense with it. I was able to adjust him and his adjustments held better. Since then life has settled down for Tomasz. He has gone on to study out of town. Now I see him only occasionally with a rare and minor complaint. I believe chiropractic care helped him through a very trying time. I wonder how many other children with a developing curvature of the spine needing a brace have to go through such pain without the help of a chiropractor. Also another question I ponder is, "Would Tomasz's scoliosis have developed as badly if he had been under chiropractic care from childhood?" By now, you know what my answer is!

Care Plan:

Tomasz started off with three visits a week, then twice a week, and currently comes once a month when it is possible.

My Little Red Car

Name: .... Milena Donovan
From: .... Mississauga,
Ontario
Treated for: .... Hip Pain;
Numbness in Feet;
Neck Stiffness;

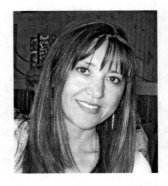

Connection Story

"My beautiful new red, convertible Mustang sports car with Shelby striping was the cause of me making an appointment with Dr. Côté last summer. All of a sudden I was beginning to have pain in my hips, either one side or the other. It was uncomfortable for me to sit and when I got up there was a cracking noise. Getting out of bed was rather nasty. I went to a medical doctor who gave me a muscle relaxant but no real relief occurred.

One day I was talking with one of the ladies at my gym who recommended chiropractic. I had been to a chiropractor years before; the neck cracking always stressed me out. My friend commented that her chiropractor, Dr. Côté, used a different method so I gave her a call.

Upon examination I learned that my one leg was ¾ of an inch shorter than the other. This could have stemmed from a number of activities. I do remember I had fallen once. Sitting in my Mustang in a "v" position with my legs raised probably aggravated my body. I finally had some validation for my pain; Dr. Côté didn't just brush me off and that was comforting. She could see there was an actual issue as a result of her x-rays and tests that she took.

After having adjustments three times a week for a period of time we did see improvement; although it did take a while before I began to really feel good again. She has also helped me with stiffness in my neck.

In the last couple of years my daughter has started playing hockey which means soreness in her back from lugging her huge hockey bag and sleeping in hotels on beds that are not so great. Dr. Côté's adjustments improve her back when it goes out of whack. Also my husband has suffered from numbness in his feet. Medical doctors have done every test possible coming up with no real answers. Dr. Côté has provided more relief to him than anyone else has. I have recommended her services to others but many are scared of hearing the sound of neck cracking as I was.

It is really wonderful that chiropractic can help in so many areas. Unfortunately, it is sad that recently we had to get rid of our little Mustang."

Comments:

Milena was an interesting case because in addition to chiropractic care to realign her femur, we had to change some of her activities as they were a big part causing her hip misalignment. She liked to work out and some of her hip stretches would force the hip out of place.

We had to discuss proper hip mechanics while "walking" which seems pretty basic but can be altered if someone is in pain long enough. I also found that sitting stretches are very hard on a weak pelvis or hip as they can force these bones out of alignment.

All this happens while you think you are doing something good for yourself and your next visit to the chiropractor's office tells you otherwise. On her last visit Milena's hips were good. During her next appointment we will be measuring her progress with my Surface Electromyography equipment.

Care Plan:

Milena came three times a week initially and is currently on a maintenance program.

I'm Fine Thank You

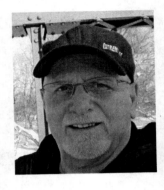

Name: .... Gary Carter
From: .... Brampton, Ontario
Treated for: .... Lower Back Pain;
Wrist Pain;
Shoulder Pain

"I'm glad I took the advice even though I
didn't believe I had a problem. It was a
long time ago when I previously had visited
a chiropractor. I assumed that the only time
to go to a chiropractor was when I
couldn't stand the back pain. And I wasn't in great pain at the current
time so I thought any advice to visit a chiropractor was misguided,
even perhaps bordering on insult. My family doctor just shrugged off
the fact that I had a little back pain from time to time. He mentioned a
common back pain drug as the remedy. I didn't need any more advice.

A friend from my wife's office talked about the great results with a
chiropractor who used a new painless technique. Because I'm curious, I
agreed to have an initial consultation. I enjoyed the visit with Dr. Côté
that day. And even though the dull ache in my back was something I
had learned to live with I was amazed as to how much better I felt
after even one adjustment. I was introduced to the Activator which
was new to me but, as I learned, has been around for quite a while. My
friend was right. It didn't hurt a bit. In fact, I wasn't even sure I had
been adjusted at first. Then the next day things were so much better.
Subsequent maintenance visits kept me feeling better than I had for 30
years.

Dr. Côté mentioned to me once that if I ever had a car accident I
should see her first. On the very day I had a front end collision and
hurt my right leg, I got in to see her. After several visits with a treatment plan she got the bones in my foot and leg property realigned. I
am so glad I discovered such a great chiropractor to help after a near
death experience.

As I look forward to the rest of my life I realize that chiropractic
maintenance with Dr. Côté is going to make a big difference to me. I
no longer dread long trips in the car. I can walk fair distances without
ending in discomfort. I can even play a little ball with the grandchildren.
And my "mouse arm" stays in place without the wrist pain I used to
bear.

I expect the quality of my life to stay at a very high level, especially in terms of my mobility. I'm approaching the age where my friends are getting orthotics, braces, knee replacements and all sorts of treatment for aches and pains. I am sure that if they took my advice and visited Dr. Côté they would have far less to worry about as the years go by. I look and feel about ten years younger than I am. I believe Dr. Côté has been a significant factor to keep me moving at a full pace. I am very grateful I didn't stick to my old view but took a friend's good advice."

Comments:

I saw Gary initially for reasons I would like to see most patients for – to maintain good health. Sure he had occasional lower back pain that he described as normal and after an initial exam realized that his posture and mobility were just a bit off the mark.

I explained what was showing and he started chiropractic care that day. He responded very quickly to the adjustments and was on a monthly schedule in a few months. The adjustments were so effective I think in part because he was not in a lot of pain and there was less muscle guarding that would prevent a quick response.

After his car accident a few years ago, Gary had more foot pain than the neck pain which we usually see. (I guess he does things a bit differently than the average person.) He didn't remember jamming his foot during the collision but misalignments were found. A bone named the talus in particular was a problem. Now Gary's foot problem is a thing of the past because he had it looked at right away.

He occasionally gets some right shoulder pain when he is on his computer too much but again he responds very well to chiropractic adjustments. I think taking care of problems at their onset rather than after years of suffering has worked wonderfully in his favour.

Care Plan:

Gary came three times a week, then once a week and now visits once every six weeks unless a new problem arises.

Three Peas in a Pod

Name: .... Sara Burton
From: .... Brampton, Ontario
Treated for: .... Tummy Aches;
Overlapped Toes;
Headaches; Knee
Pain; Indigestion

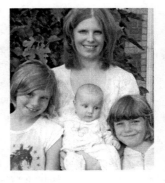

"As a fitness professional I have always felt the benefit of chiropractic for myself. Chiropractic has helped me stay away from injury and I just feel better with regular adjustments. When my third child was born, my mother recommended that I take her to see Dr. Côté. I decided to take all three girls for a general check-up.

In the waiting room I started to fill out all the appropriate paperwork and realized how many things I needed to have Dr. Côté assess.

We began with Kaiya. As she started assessing I mentioned that she was having tummy aches and we couldn't identify what was causing them. I had not thought of asking the chiropractor about this but stomach problems was on the questionnaire so what was there to lose. Within a few minutes Dr. Côté saw that one of her lower ribs was out of place and that could be the cause. I then asked her to look at her toes as they tended to crunch up together where her second toe sat on top of her big toe. My mouth dropped open when she stood up in front of me after her adjustment and all five toes were lined up perfectly in a row.

Cassidy was next and one thing I knew I had to mention was that she was experiencing headaches at least once or twice every month. As Dr. Côté lifted her feet up we could all see that one side was showing significantly shorter. One click of the activator to her neck, she checked again and the two shoes lined up perfectly. That would explain the headaches if her C2 was so out. She continued her assessment and found something misaligned in her lower leg. Later we learned that her knee was hurting her but she hadn't mentioned it. Dr. Côté was able to realign it even before we realized it.

Finally she took a look at the baby. Again I could clearly see how when Carleigh extended both of her legs, one was shorter. Dr. Côté then asked if we had any problems with a whole list of things and – yep, spitting up! She had me hold the baby this way, then that. One click to the T12, one to the atlas and she was completely balanced.

I was completely impressed with the precision Dr. Côté used. She listened to what I had to say and spent a significant amount of time studying and assessing that any manipulations she did were quick and clearly accurate. I had never been an observer of a chiropractor, but what I saw gave me hope that we would be able to more quickly and effectively address the issues we were simply just dealing with. Thank you Dr. Côté!"

Comments:

Adjusting kids is extremely rewarding for a chiropractor as they respond faster and more dramatically than adults do. I have seen children with all kinds of ailments in the last 25 years – from colic to ear infections, from asthma (my son being one of them) to ADD. There is always an improvement in the condition when their structure is better aligned.

Children seem to know innately that the adjustments are good for them even when they are infants. As they get older some will even ask me themselves for an adjustment if they are in with their parents and not scheduled that day. They know they will be better afterwards.

Care Plan:

Since most kids do react quickly I schedule them for a few visits close together to see how the alignments hold and to observe their response. Then sometimes I will decrease the number of visits gradually to once a month or even once every three months depending on the health of the child.

A Bleary-Eyed Goalie Isn't a Good Thing

Name: .... Joe Amlinger
From: .... Elmira, Ontario
Treated for: ..... shoulder pain, blurred vision

Connection Story

My family and Dr. Côté along with her family have been good friends all my life. My father is a chiropractor as well so I learned the importance of being adjusted regularly from an early age. "Auntie Miche" would even bring her Activator instrument along with her when we vacationed together.

In 2006, my second year of university, I played goalie for my hockey team. I began to notice that my vision would grow bleary. I couldn't even see the numbers on the scoreboard. I had never worn glasses or contact lenses. With my busy school life I didn't think much of it but eventually I decided it was time to have things checked out. I had been experiencing problems with my shoulder so I called up Dr. Côté in Mississauga. She let me come over to her house right away for an adjustment. I was really out of alignment and so I continued to see her once a week for a while. During the following summer I returned home and didn't play hockey until I went back to school in the fall. My eyesight was fine at that point until closer to Christmas my vision started getting blurry once more which signaled I needed another adjustment.

My family and I have since moved to Elmira, ON and I am seeing a chiropractor recommended by Dr. Côté on a regular basis – no matter what. I definitely recommend chiropractic to others.

Comments:

Whenever I would see Joe for an emergency visit, his blurred vision would promptly return to normal. I attribute his quick recoveries to his lifelong chiropractic care as his father is a chiropractor. He has been adjusted regularly from birth.

There have been many accounts of eyesight improvement with chiropractic care but it is only recently that scientific data is emerging to tabulate these types of results. One study in particular authored by Dr. Chanhjiang reported on 114 cases of patients with cervical spine problems who had visual disorders. Improvement in vision was noted in 83% of these cases after receiving "manipulative treatment."[16] Dr. AGJ Terrett, a chiropractor, suggests that "... brain and retinal cells are thought to "hibernate" when in a state of relative ischemia (lack of oxygen). Such an ischemic state does not kill the cells, but renders them incapable of normal function. Upon restoration of normal blood supply, the improved oxygenation of the involved cells may restore normal function."[17]

Care Plan:

Being away at university I saw Joe only occasionally when his vision was significantly disturbed. We never did set a specific care plan in place for him. It is, however, interesting to document his experience because vision problems are not usually associated with chiropractic. Sometimes even one chiropractic adjustment can prove to be priceless.

Thought to Ponder:

**If ignorance is bliss,
why aren't people happier?**

**"Life is what we make it: always has
been, always will be."**

Grandma Moses

9

Final Thoughts

How a Sincere Health Care Professional Makes a Difference

Many of my family members chose the wonderful health care profession called chiropractic. I am proud of the start my father gave me. His brother Roger was also a chiropractor. My husband and his brother followed their father's footsteps as well. I guess when you observe someone close to you doing something they are passionate about, it's easy to want to achieve the same.

College Daze

One of the biggest misconceptions about chiropractic is that you become one because you couldn't qualify for enrolling in a medical school.

The truth is that it is not easy to enter the college in Toronto where I attended or any chiropractic college. The entrance requirement is a three or four year Bachelor of Science degree. Above average marks are needed to enroll. The hours of study and the subjects taught are almost identical to that of a medical school. This education cannot be considered a short cut; a chiropractic student works just as hard, covers the same material and spends a lot more on tuition.

For example, one study in the U.S. compared the curriculum of 22 medical schools and 11 chiropractic colleges. Based on the overall average, chiropractic students invest 13% more classroom time than the medical doctor students. There are several areas where the medical students spend more time, such as in chemistry, psychiatry and obstetrics. However even in these three areas the chiropractic students participate in 285 classroom hours. On the other hand, chiropractic students spend 208 more hours than the medical doctor students do studying neurology as this is what they deal with day in and day out. As you can see regarding education the doctor of chiropractic and the medical doctor are on equal footing.

After learning and practicing in an outpatient clinic connected with my college, I took oral and written exams. Upon graduation at the college ceremony we pledged the following Chiropractic Oath, as chiropractors before and after me have done. This oath helps us keep in mind the incisive comment made by Hippocrates, known as the Father of medicine, "Look well to the spine for the cause of disease."

And I Mean It

"I do hereby swear before God and these assembled witnesses, both corporeal and spiritual, that I will do my utmost to keep this, my sacred, trusted oath, as a graduate of Canadian Memorial Chiropractic College, that henceforth:

I will esteem those who taught me this Art, Science and Philosophy of Chiropractic and with this torch fashioned by Hippocrates, I will light the way to the understanding of those Natural Laws which preserve the human body as a fitting temple for the soul of man.

I will keep the physical, mental and spiritual needs of the sick as my foremost duty, ever searching for and correcting the cause of their disease to the best of my ability, insofar as my science is in the highest precepts of my Alma Mater and harmonious with the Vis Medicatrix Naturae.

I will at all times stand ready to serve my fellow man, without distinction of race, creed or color, in my lifelong vocation of preventing and alleviating human suffering wherever it may be found, by exemplifying in my own life a pattern of living in harmony with the laws of nature.

I will refrain from any act of wrong doing and will regard the keeping of a patient's confidence as a moral obligation, using any such information in his or her best interests.

May God so direct the skillful use of my hands that I may bring strength to the sick, relief to the suffering, peace of mind to the anxious and the inspiration of mankind to attain bountiful health that we may live this life to the fullest expression of its innate endowments. I therefore solemnly swear to uphold those principles and precepts to the best of my ability, so help me God.''[18]

And I Still Mean It

Since that momentous day in my life, I have upheld the oath I made to the best of my ability and have continued to learn and study my field of science as do other chiropractors. About six times a year I am off to a seminar for a few days to learn about new advances in my profession including office management, inspiration, techniques, pediatrics, and CPR. I am also required to keep a professional portfolio to maintain a license and keep track of all the professional development efforts to stay current. These include professional journals read, seminars attended, professional CDs listened to etc. This ongoing education helps me keep up to date on the latest philosophies and technologies to run my practice as smoothly as possible and to pass some of that education along to my patients as well. There are some upgrades we need to do from time to time to maintain our license which are organized by our licensing board. Also our practice has to be reviewed by our peers to make sure we are doing everything possible to protect the public. All this builds my confidence in what we do as chiropractors and helps to strengthen the confidence of our patients.

If another health care professional says you should not see a chiropractor, inquire if this person has ever taken a chiropractor to lunch to discuss the various approaches they use to help their patients. Ask this health practitioner how they would account for the many personal experiences described in this book. Can they all be written off so easily? If the answers do not measure up to your satisfaction why would you take their opinion seriously? This is similar to asking for advice about purchasing a car from someone who has never owned or even driven one. Go for a second opinion!

Are You Making the Connection Yet?

Have you made the connection yet? You probably did not know why or how chiropractic can help. You have read the many stories here of people who did connect good chiropractic care with the problems they were facing. You don't have to wait until the problem is unbearable. At the first indication of a health problem, I want you to think of your chiropractor. That could save you time, money and suffering!

Every day in my practice I see patients who have come to the end of the road medically with their particular health problem. As a last resort they have ended up in my office out of desperation and feeling as if they having nothing to lose any more. When these patients realize how easy, safe and effective chiropractic care is at solving their "incurable" problem, they are thrilled that they can finally experience great health. However in the back of their minds there is also anger and frustration with not having that knowledge sooner. All the unnecessary pain and suffering, unnecessary expenses and procedures, unnecessary time wasted could have been avoided had the correct information about chiropractic been readily available. This is what motivated the creation of this book so more people can find the chiropractic answer to health problems.

Do you remember Marcus Bach, B.J. Palmer's friend, who traveled the world to find previous evidence of chiropractic? Here is his final conclusion:

"From a humble start in 1895, chiropractic grew into a world wide movement, universally accepted, and it stands today as the most formidable challenger to medicine's 5000 years of authoritarian rule. Its goal is not to unseat medicine but rather to discover and develop the most truthfully scientific method by which the sick can be made well and the well be kept from getting sick." [19]

We've got your back and so much more!

Appendix I
Health Conditions

S ince 1982 when I started my practice I have seen all kinds of problems that have responded well from the very common to sometimes the very unusual. Here are three lists of ailments seen in my practice to trigger your thinking. These lists are not complete and other chiropractors may be able to add additional conditions from their practices. Please keep in mind that it's not the scope or practice of a chiropractor to test and evaluate any of these conditions. It is the chiropractor's responsibility to test and evaluate structural misalignments that may as a consequence have an impact on the particular health issue. The chiropractor has been trained to refer a patient to another health care specialist if the condition warrants it.

Are you suffering with one of these problems? Maybe it is time to seek the help of a chiropractor.

A. Here are some of the most common conditions I have seen improve in my practice:

- Anxiety attacks
- Arm problems (e.g. weakness, pins & needles, numbness)
- Bedwetting
- Bladder infections
- Carpal Tunnel Syndrome or other wrist/hand pain
- Chest pain
- Coccyx pain or disorders
- Colds
- Constipation
- Digestive Problems
- Disc problems
- Dizziness
- Ear infections
- Facial neuralgia
- Flu
- Headaches/migraine
- Heartburn
- Hip problems

- Insomnia
- Irritable Bowel Syndrome
- Knee/leg/foot pain
- Low/mid back pain
- Menstrual cramps
- Migraine Headaches
- Nausea
- Neck pain or post whiplash neck problems
- Osteoarthritis conditions
- Plantar Fasciitis
- Pinched nerves
- Piriformis Syndrome
- Sacroiliac problems
- Sciatica
- Scoliosis
- Shoulder problems
- Stress
- TMJ disorders
- Vertigo

B. Also, I have seen these conditions often improved over longer periods of time with regular chiropractic care:

- Allergies
- Asthma
- Blood pressure problems
- Certain heart conditions
- Chronic sinusitis
- Colic
- Depression
- Disc herniations
- Eczema or skin rashes
- Hiatus Hernia
- Immune system disorders
- Indigestion
- Infertility
- Lack of energy
- Restless Leg Syndrome
- Thyroid problems

C. Here are some of the most unusual problems I have seen respond very well in my office:

*   Anger fits (uncontrolled)
*   Chronic hiccups
*   Colitis
*   Pre-gangrenous foot
*   Swelling in feet/legs
*   Tongue numbness

Keep in mind that these kinds of conditions can be caused by other problems not involving the nervous system. If that is the case, then your chiropractor can determine that from the assessment and refer you to the appropriate specialist as what happened with Kyle in Chapter 9.

Appendix II
Chiropractic Influence on Oxidative Stress and DNA Repair

There is a growing body of evidence that wellness care provided by doctors of chiropractic may reduce health care costs, improve health behaviors, and enhance patient perceived quality of life. Until recently, however, little was known about how chiropractic adjustments affected the chemistry of biological processes on a cellular level.

In a landmark study published this week in the Journal of Vertebral Subluxation Research (JVSR; www.jvsr.com), chiropractors collaborating with researchers at the University of Lund found that chiropractic care could influence basic physiological processes affecting oxidative stress and DNA repair. These findings offer a scientific explanation for the positive health benefits reported by patients receiving chiropractic care.

The researchers measured serum thiol levels in 21 patients under short-term chiropractic care and 25 patients under long-term chiropractic care. The results were compared to those of a non-chiropractic treated control group of 30 subjects. Long-term chiropractic care of two or more years was shown to reestablish a normal physiological state independent of age, sex, or nutritional supplements. Symptom-free or primary wellness subjects under chiropractic care demonstrated higher mean serum thiol levels than patients with active disease, and produced some values that were higher than normal wellness values.

Serum thiols are primary antioxidants, and serve as a measure of human health status. The test provides a surrogate estimate of DNA repair enzyme activity, which has been shown to correlate with lifespan and aging.

Dr. Christopher Kent, one of the authors explained, "Going through life, we experience physical, chemical, and emotional stress. These stresses affect the function of the nervous system. We hypothesized that these disturbances in nerve function could affect oxidative stress and DNA repair on a cellular level."

"Oxidative stress, metabolically generating free radicals, is now a broadly accepted theory of how we age and develop disease," Kent continued. "Oxidative stress results in DNA damage, and inhibits DNA repair. DNA repair is the mechanism which fixes the damage caused by environmental impact."

Chiropractors apply spinal adjustments to correct disturbances of nerve function. "Chiropractic care appears to improve the ability of the body to adapt to stress," continued Kent. "Further research is needed to gain additional insights that will ultimately lead to improved clinical outcomes," he said.

The study was a collaborative involving Camgen, Inc. of Victoria, B.C. Canada; Chiropractic Leadership Alliance in Mahwah, NJ; Biomedical Diagnostic Research, LLC in Chesterland, Ohio; and Department of Cell and Molecular Biology of Tumor Immunology, University of Lund, Sweden.

JVSR is a peer-reviewed scientific journal devoted to subluxation-based chiropractic research affiliated with the World Chiropractic Alliance (WCA), an international organization representing doctors of chiropractic. WCA promotes the traditional, drug-free and non-invasive form of chiropractic as a means of correcting vertebral subluxations that cause nerve interference.

World Chiropractic Alliance (WCA)
Chandler, AZ 85224
United States
Phone 800-347-1011

www.worldchiropracticalliance.org

End Notes

1 Philip Yancy, Dr. Paul Brand, *The Gift of Pain* (Grand Rapids, Michigan: Zondervan Publishing House, 1993) p. 5.

2 *Britannica Online Encyclopedia,* www.Britannica.com.

3 *Merriam-Webster Online Dictionary,* www.merriam-webster.com, 2008.

4 *Cambridge Online Dictionary,*www.dictionary.cambridge.org.

5 Dr. J. David Cassidy,*Seven-Year Neck Pain Study Sheds Light on Best Care* (Bone and Joint Decade Task Force - Press Release, February 2008.)

6 Marcus Bach, *The Chiropractic Story* (Los Angeles, CA: DeVorss & Co., Inc., 1968) p. 25.

7 Ibid., p. 26.

8 Ibid., p. 41.

9 Ibid., p. 89-90.

10 Ibid., p. 246.

11 Ibid., p. 166.

12 Katie Gilbert, *Immune Boost: This is Spinal Zap* (Psychology Today, August 24, 2006).

13 W. Heath Quigley, *Clear View Sanitarium – Unforgettable Personalities* (Dynamic Chiropractic, Vol. 8 - Issue 6, March 14, 1990).

14 Arlan W. Fuhr, *Activator Methods – Chiropractic Technique* (Mosby – Year Book Inc., 1997). p. 8.

15 Pran Manga & Assoc. Inc., *Manga Report Executive Summary – The Effectiveness and Cost-Effectiveness of Chiropractic Management of Low-Back Pain,* 1993.

16 Changjiang I, Yici W, Wenquin L, et al: *"Study on cervical visual disturbance and its manipulative treatment."* Journal of Traditional Chinese Medicine 1984 4:205.

17 AGJ Terrett, *"Cerebral dysfunction: a theory to explain some of the effects of chiropractic spinal manipulation."* Chiropractic Technique (1993) 5(4):168.

18 Robert Dryburgh, *So You're Thinking of Going to a Chiropractor,* (New Canaan, Connecticut: Keats Publishing, Inc., 1984) p. 127-128.

19 Bach, *The Chiropractic Story,* p. 246-247.

Index

CPSIA information can be obtained at www.ICGtesting.com
Printed in the USA
BVOW02s2218230114

342895BV00010B/472/P